Healthy Vegetatian Cookbook

2 Books in 1 Plant-Based Diet for, Vegan Meal Prep

By Michael Garavaglia

form the information ultimately takes. This includes copied versions of the work both physical, digital and audio unless express consent of the Publisher is provided beforehand. Any additional rights reserved.

Furthermore, the information that can be found within the pages described forthwith shall be considered both accurate and truthful when it comes to the recounting of facts. As such, any use, correct or incorrect, of the provided information will render the Publisher free of responsibility as to the actions taken outside of their direct purview. Regardless, there are zero scenarios where the original author or the Publisher can be deemed liable in any fashion for any damages or hardships that may result from any of the information discussed herein.

Additionally, the information in the following pages is intended only for informational purposes and should thus be thought of as universal. As befitting its nature, it is presented without assurance regarding its prolonged validity or interim quality. Trademarks that are mentioned are done without written consent and can in no way be considered an endorsement from the trademark holder.

BOOK 1

Plant-Based Diet for Weight Loss

The Paradox of an Introductory Guide on How to Kill Bad Habits so as not to Die of Fat (50 Delicious Bonus Recipes for the Vegetable-Based Diet)

By Michael Garavaglia

form the information ultimately takes. This includes copied versions of the work both physical, digital and audio unless express consent of the Publisher is provided beforehand. Any additional rights reserved.

Furthermore, the information that can be found within the pages described forthwith shall be considered both accurate and truthful when it comes to the recounting of facts. As such, any use, correct or incorrect, of the provided information will render the Publisher free of responsibility as to the actions taken outside of their direct purview. Regardless, there are zero scenarios where the original author or the Publisher can be deemed liable in any fashion for any damages or hardships that may result from any of the information discussed herein.

Additionally, the information in the following pages is intended only for informational purposes and should thus be thought of as universal. As befitting its nature, it is presented without assurance regarding its prolonged validity or interim quality. Trademarks that are mentioned are done without written consent and can in no way be considered an endorsement from the trademark holder.

Table of Contents

Chapter 7: 10 Dessert Recipes

Chapter 8: Starting Your Weight Loss Program: A Four-Week Plan

Chapter 1: Introduction to Plant-Based Eating

The Importance of a Plant-based Diet for your Body and Health

The vegan diet or plant-based way of eating is a great way to improve your health and lifestyle by replacing all animal products and by-products with easy-to-digest plant-based foods. Following a plant-based diet has grown in popularity and is embraced by a lot of people, including celebrities, chefs, and ordinary people from all backgrounds. Some cultures embrace vegan meals and have for centuries, long before plant-based eating become more mainstream and available to everyone. There are many health benefits from switching to a vegan diet:

1. Weight loss is one of the major benefits of a plant-based diet. Many studies and research indicate that a diet without animal fats and protein is low in fat and contributes to lower rates of obesity, and on average, a healthier weight. This is due to the high fiber and low amount of fat in many fruits, vegetables, and other plant-based foods.

2. There is a high level of nutrients in a plant-based diet, as
   the foods include a wide variety of fruits and vegetables
   which contain numerous vitamins, minerals,
   antioxidants, and calcium. Certain vegetables contain a
   lot of protein, such as dark leafy greens kale, spinach, and
   arugula. Focusing on more varieties of plant-based foods
   can increase the number of nutrients in your diet.

3. Prevention of cancer is another benefit of a plant-based
   diet. Some research shows promising results on how
   changing to a vegan diet can prevent and reverse some
   forms of cancer. A high number of antioxidants, found in
   fresh fruits and vegetables, are responsible for slowing
   the formation of free radicals, which contribute to
   cancerous cell growth and other debilitating diseases and
   conditions. There is a lower rate of cancer among plant-
   based eaters, which is a good reason to ditch the meat.

4. Lower rates of heart disease and better blood pressure are
   benefits of a vegan diet, due to the lack of animal fats,
   which contribute to high blood pressure and clogged
   arteries, especially when consumed regularly. The
   elimination of meat increases heart health and helps
   prevent many chronic and more serious conditions that

can result from high blood pressure and related heart conditions.

5. Chronic conditions such as arthritis and fibromyalgia can be devastating for many people, though there are specific nutrients such as vitamin A and C can alleviate symptoms of these conditions and prevent inflammation and related pain that can result. Many fruits and vegetables contain anti-inflammatory properties that are beneficial for many conditions, by reducing pain and swelling.

6. Regulating insulin levels and maintaining healthy blood sugar levels are great benefits of the vegan diet. Fruits contain sugar, though the amount is enough for a healthy diet and is easily digested by the body, whereas refined and artificial forms of sugar contribute to high glucose levels, which increase the risk of Type 2 Diabetes.

7. Plant-based eaters often report higher levels of energy, which makes it easier to stay active, exercise and keep weight at a reasonable level.

8. A vegan diet can improve the health of skin, nails, and hair by reducing the number of blemishes and breakouts.

9. In some cases, vegan diets can be less expensive and easier to shop for than diets that include meat, fish, and dairy products, which are often costly. Beans, grains, legumes, nuts, and seeds, all of which are plant-based and full of nutrients, can be purchased in bulk and enjoyed in small amounts as an important part of your eating plan.

10. Plant-based eating can help alleviate many other conditions, including high cholesterol, digestive conditions, and nutrient deficiencies. Due to contrary belief, a vegan diet can meet all your nutrient requirements, including B12 and vitamin D.

Exploring new foods and recipes is an excellent way to adapt to a plant-based diet, which doesn't need to occur overnight. It's best to gradually introduce new foods into the diet and discover which ones you like the best for future menu and meal planning. Often, people focus on dietary restrictions, instead of enjoying the amount of flexibility and new opportunities many foods provide. A plant-based diet is a scientifically proven healthy way to eat and enjoy food for a lifetime, and you'll love the benefits it provides!

The Impact of Eating Processed Foods and Meat on Weight Gain and Disease

Many people enjoy a wider variety of foods on a vegan diet. This is not just because they are simply replacing meat and dairy products, but rather, focusing on the wide range of foods that are plant-based. Over time, you'll notice some major improvements to your health and well-being, which includes losing excess weight and improving your metabolism. Meat products may seem like a good choice in dieting, especially when choosing lean meats and fish. However, there are a lot of pesticides and chemicals used in processing meats that can impact our bodies and how we digest them. There are also growing concerns about the treatment of animals in factory farming and how this impacts their lives as well as ours. Choosing vegan not only makes a healthier lifestyle but a more ethical one as well.

Chapter 2: How to Start a New Diet Plan and Ditch Unhealthy Habits

Focus on Plant-Based Proteins and Nutrients

Choosing the right plant-based protein for your diet is easier than you think, and there are more options than most people realize. Many of the common vegetable proteins on the market tend to be more versatile and available in a variety of forms and textures, which makes adding them to your diet effortless. In fact, there is a much wider range of plant-based protein than animal-based.

Soy Products

One of the most popular and commonly purchased vegan proteins is soy. Tofu, tempeh, miso, soymilk, and other dairy-free products are included in this category. Tempeh and miso are fermented forms of soy and contain B12, calcium, protein, and fiber. They are excellent additions to any meal, including soups, stir fry dishes, roasts, and salads. Tofu remains a common option for vegans and contains a high amount of both protein and calcium. Soy-based drinks and dairy replacements are often soy-based, such as yogurts, creams, cheese, and milk.

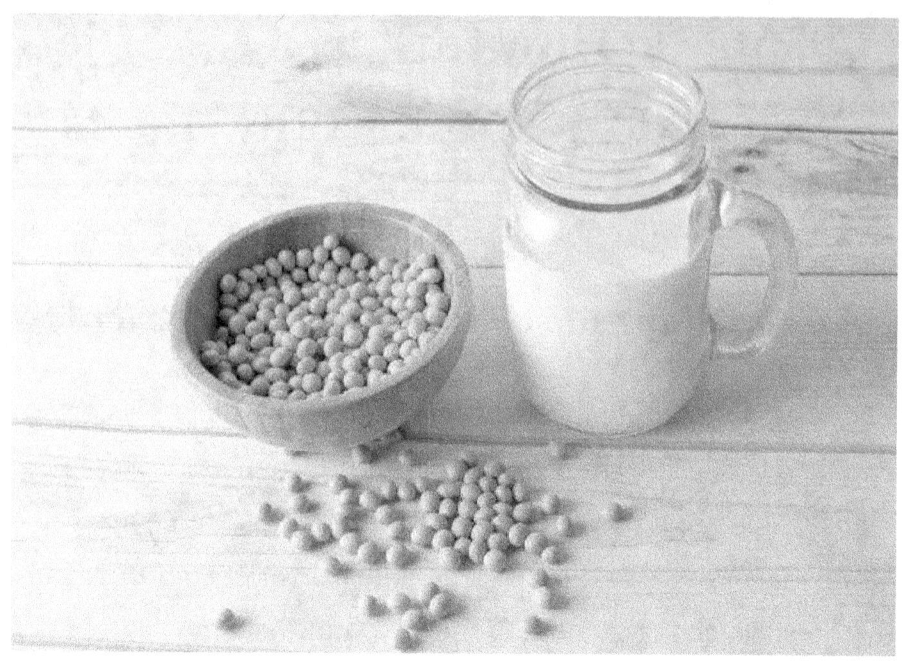

Seitan

This protein source is made from gluten, which is found in whole wheat. It is a form of protein that is made by isolating the gluten or protein content from the wheat. This process of making seitan is usually time-consuming, and not often the most commonly used vegan protein, though it is a good option for people with soy allergies. Seitan should be avoided by people who are gluten intolerant. It can be found in some natural food stores.

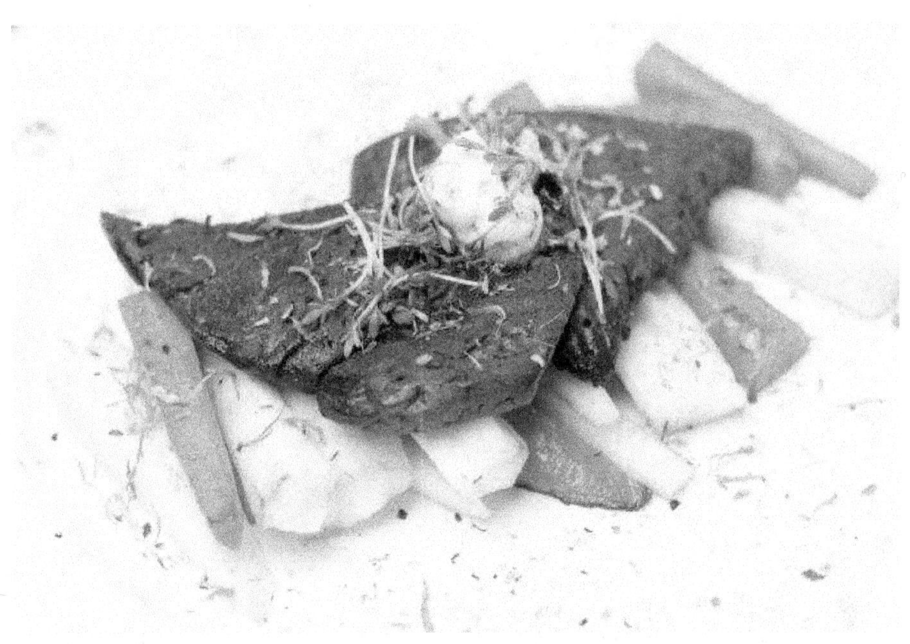

Lentils

These beans are easy to cook and don't require the soaking time that kidney beans, chickpeas, black beans, and other varieties require. They are flavorful and can be easily added to soups, stews, and salads. On their own, they can create tasty dishes full of spice.

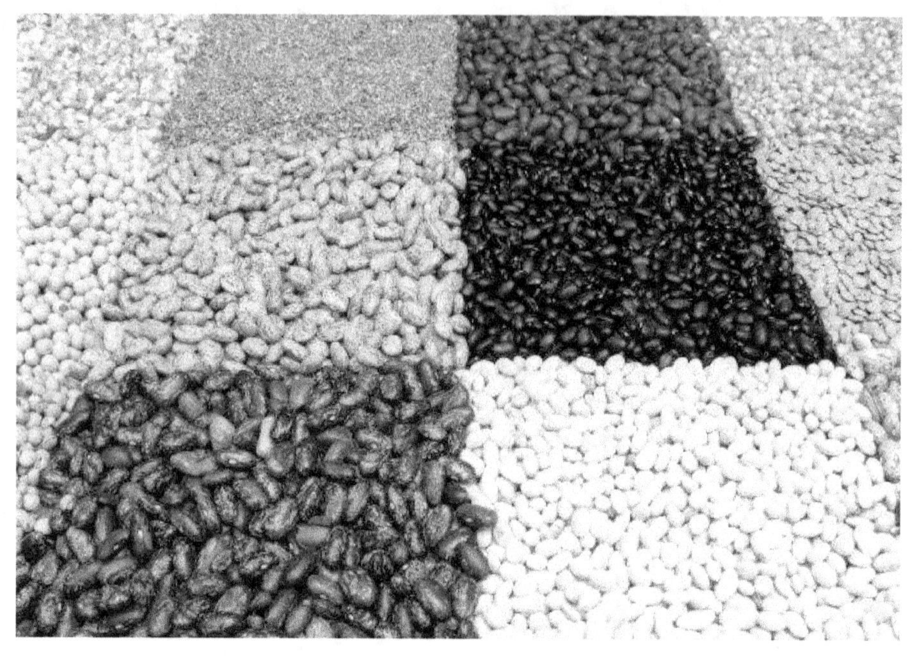

Chickpeas

A good source of protein and fiber, chickpeas are always good to have in the pantry for many soups, salads, and stews. Canned or dried, chickpeas are inexpensive and easy to add to a variety of meals

<u>*Quinoa*</u>

It's often considered both a grain and a pulse. Quinoa is a high-protein food with amino acids that can take the place of rice and other sides in many dishes. It's a great side dish on its own, or as a supplement to stews and soups. Many salads add quinoa to boost the fiber and protein content.

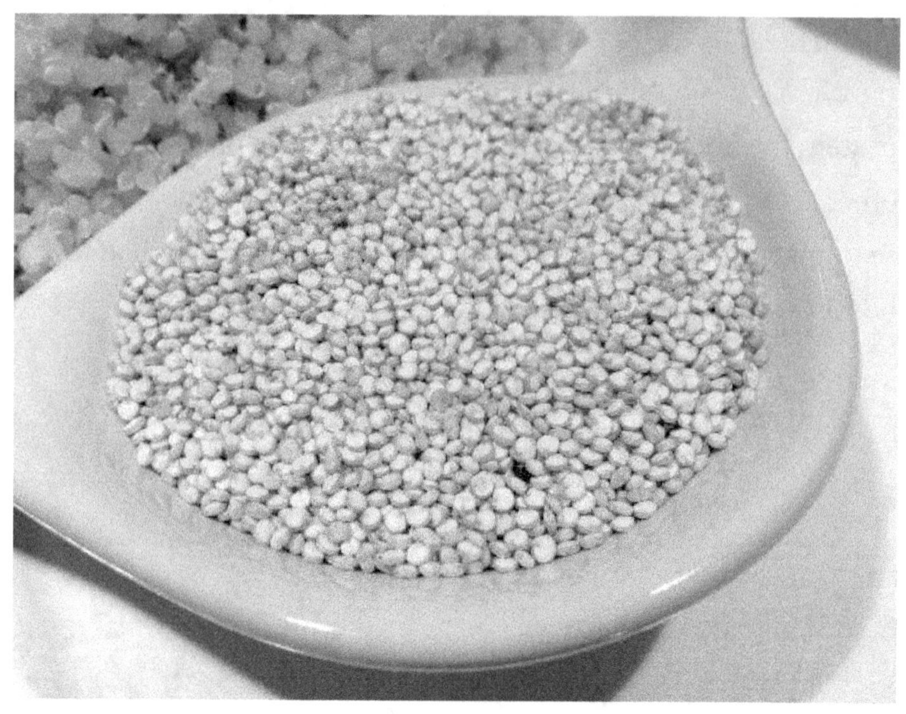

Green Peas

A sweet, flavorful vegetable, green peas are a good protein source. They are also high in fiber and make a pleasant ingredient in soups and baked dishes, such as shepherd's pie and other casseroles.

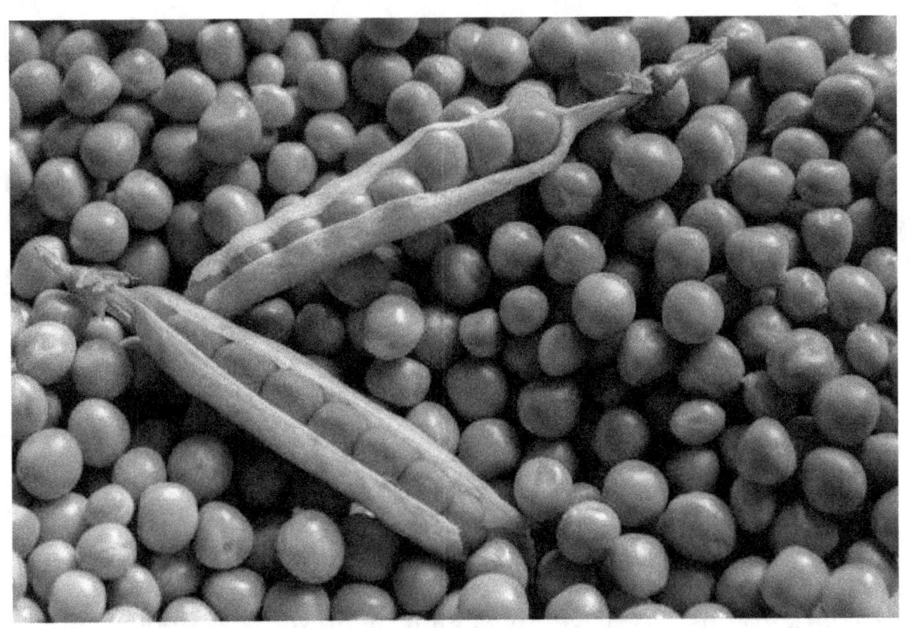

Foods to Choose for Your Diet: Keeping it Healthy and Vegan

Creating a shopping list can be a challenging experience when there are changes to your diet or the need to work within budgetary constraints. When choosing plant-based foods, concentrate on the fresh produce and natural foods as much as possible, avoiding packaged and artificially flavored options. This is especially important for ensuring you get the most nutrients possible while having access to a variety of choices. The following selection of items provides a good start for building your shopping list.

Fresh (and Frozen) Produce Section

This section of the grocery store is located around the perimeters of the store and contains the bulk of items you'll need for your shopping trip. Most stores contain a good variety of options, and wherever possible, it's best to choose fruits and vegetables in season, as they are fresh and locally harvested. If there are specific fruits or vegetables unavailable in the produce section, they may be found in the frozen section. Frozen is the next best option after fresh, and if neither is an option, choose canned.

Dark leafy greens are one of the most highly nutritious vegetables you can include in your diet, and are especially important for vegans, due to the high calcium and fiber content. Kale, arugula, and spinach are among the most nutrient-rich in the dark greens. For vegetables high in vitamin C, choose bell peppers. Onions and garlic are also useful for flavoring a wide variety of meals, as well as dried or fresh herbs and spices. Cabbage, green peas, carrots, squash, potatoes, and yams are among some of the best vegetables for creating a lot of meals, and they tend to be inexpensive and readily available in most stores.

Citrus fruits are a good source of vitamin C, while berries are high in antioxidants in general. Apples and bananas make excellent snacks on their own, because of their portability: they are already "packaged" in their skin and can be taken on the go for convenient snacking anywhere. Pomegranates and avocados are especially rich in vitamins and should be considered when they are available, even if you only purchase one or two.

Soy Products and Dairy Alternatives

During your shopping trip, you'll notice the tofu, sprouts, and many meat-free and dairy alternatives are located close to (or right in) the produce section. This is a convenient location for combining your vegetable proteins with your grocery selection. Tofu is usually available in a variety of flavors, alongside tempeh and an array of dairy-free cheeses, "meat" balls, patties, and sausages. Miso paste is usually available in this area, or where other soups can be found.

Sprouts, herbs, and spices

These can be purchased dry or fresh. If you choose fresh, make sure they are used quickly to avoid wilting. Sprouts must also be used within a day or so in order to keep the freshness and quality of nutrients available. Some stores offer these products in bulk, which can be helpful if you only require a small portion at a time.

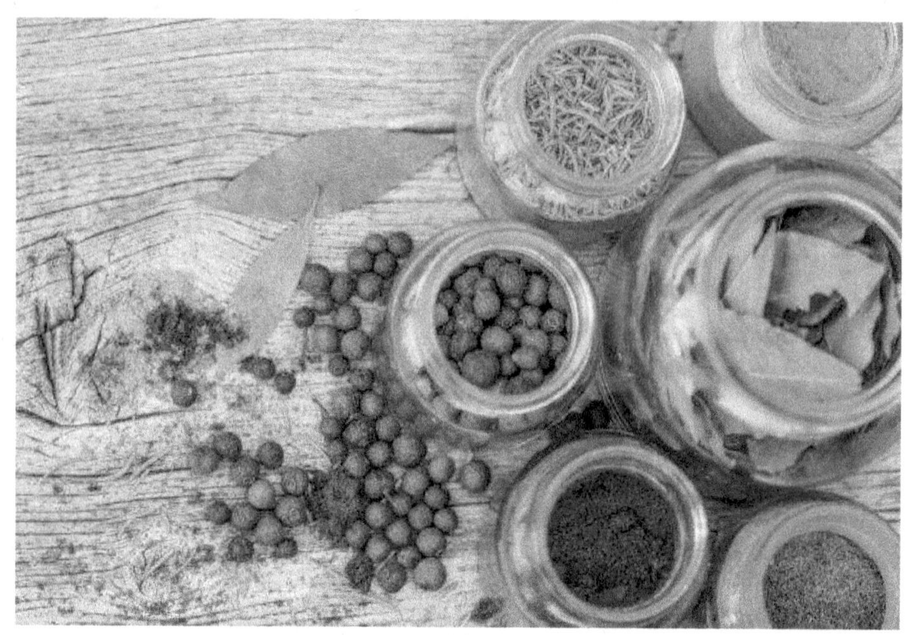

Nuts and Seeds

Pumpkin, sesame, chia, flax, and hemp seeds are all high in protein, fatty acids, and vitamins. Chia seeds are the most nutrient-dense of these seeds and can be found in natural food stores, as well as many regular grocery stores. Nuts are a good snack and topping or addition to many dishes. These can be found in the bulk aisle or close to the snack section. Most people skip these foods, not realizing their potential.

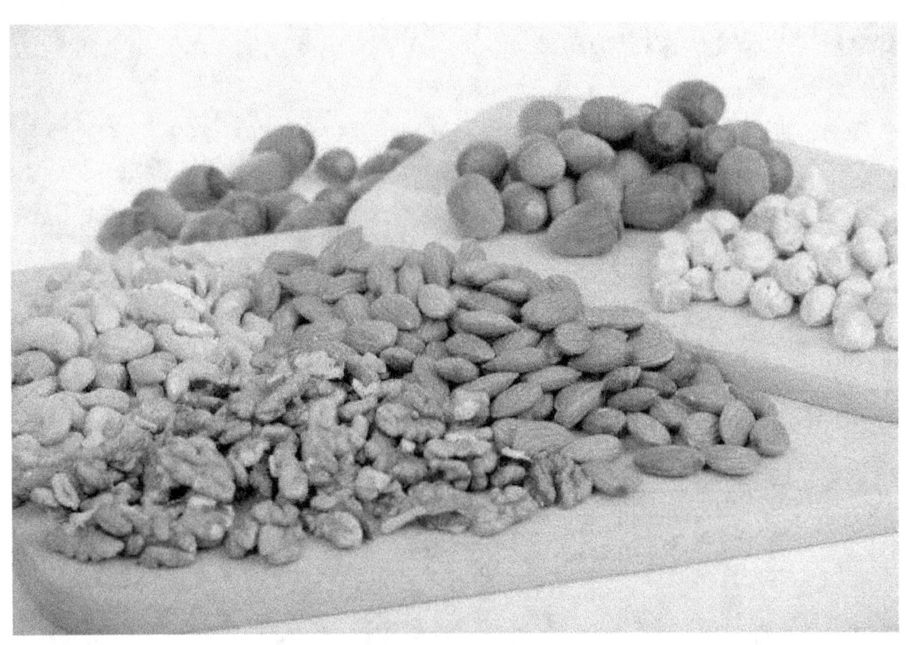

Diary-Free Milk and Vegan Alternatives to Dairy Products

Soymilk is the most common and frequently used non-dairy beverage, though there are a growing number of other options, including coconut, hazelnut, rice, and almond milk. Hemp and oats milk are also options in some natural food stores. Dairy-free yogurt, cheese, sour cream, and butter are often found in the dairy section and/or with the assortment of tofu and other plant-based options in the produce section.

Shopping for a plant-based diet means avoiding some key areas around the grocery store or market, as well as many foods that are not suitable or healthy. Some vegan foods can be unhealthy if they contain a lot of preservatives or artificial ingredients, such as some packaged vegan "meats" and cheeses. It's best to use your own discretion to determine which options work best for you.

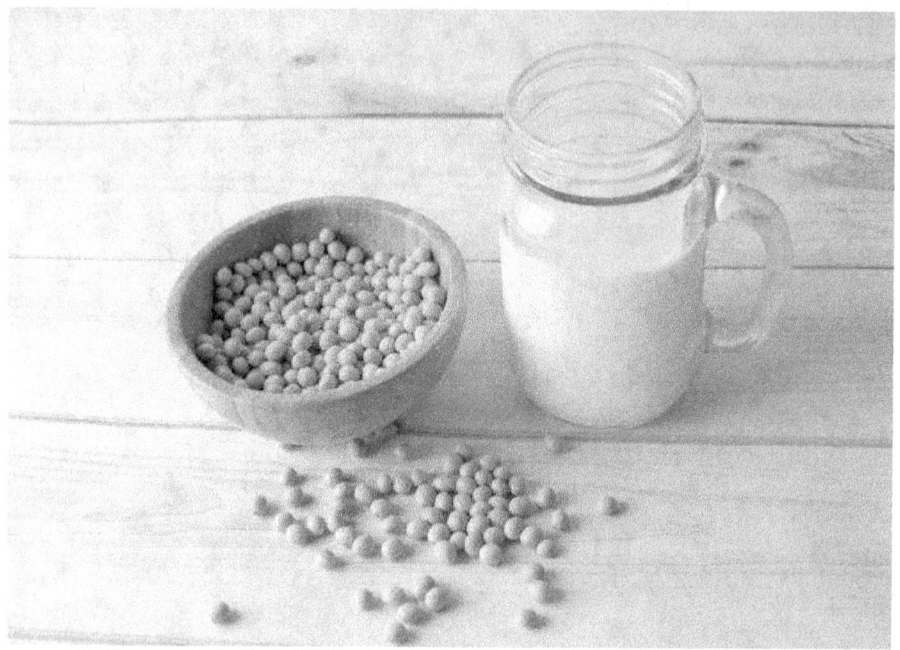

Foods to Avoid on a Vegan Diet

The following foods are best to avoid on a vegan diet, whether they are animal-based, meat by-products, or simply not a good choice for optimal health and weight loss:

- Flavored, processed vegan "meats", such as faux sausages, burgers, and cheeses with a lot of artificial ingredients. Some are better options than others, which can be researched and determined ahead of your next shopping trip

- Meat and dairy products. With the exception of some soy-based and dairy-free milk and related items located in the dairy section, all other foods should be skipped, including meats, dairy, and eggs.

- Sugary and high sodium snacks are best to avoid, as they can be easily replaced with nuts, seeds, and fresh fruits.

- Soda and fruit juice are high in sugar and will work against your efforts to lose weight and keep it off. For this reason, avoid these drinks altogether, and choose sparkling water (with natural flavor), coffee, tea, and water.

- Ice cream is another option that should be avoided, although there are some vegan options that can serve as a treat on occasion.

- Baked goods, bread, and cakes should generally be avoided unless you are aware of dairy-free bread or baked foods are options. Pastries and other sweet bakery treats are best to avoid because of their high sugar content. Some bakeries feature vegan baking, which can be a nice indulgence on occasion.

Make a list of grocery items and/or categories of the foods you want to include in your next shopping trip to make the task much easier. You'll find that shopping vegan is much easier, as you will only need to focus your attention on certain areas of the store. It may seem to limit at first, however, once you observe the full range of foods and options within these categories, you may be tempted to try new foods and flavors you may never have considered before, making your shopping experience more of an adventure.

Chapter 3: 10 Easy Smoothies for Breakfast

Breakfast Smoothies for a quick breakfast on the go. They provide a good portion of nutrients, many of which meet our body's daily requirements. There are many options for plant-based smoothies, including a wide range of fruits, non-dairy milk options, sweeteners, and spices. The best options for sweeteners are maple syrup and low carb options, such as swerve and monk fruit.

Avocado Banana Smoothie

This is a nutrient-rich smoothie that works to give you an abundance of energy and fiber in one serving. The combination of bananas and avocado provides a good serving of protein, healthy fats, potassium, and antioxidants. The milk used in this recipe is coconut due to its thick consistency, which creates a creamy texture, though almond and other nut milk are good choices as well.

- 1 ripe avocado

- 1 banana

- 2 cups of coconut milk (or another dairy-free option)

- 2 tablespoons of natural sweetener

- ½ cups of ice

Blend the milk, avocado, and banana together, then add in the sweetener and pulse briefly. Ice can be added and crushed to chill before serving. Makes two servings. The preparation time is five minutes.

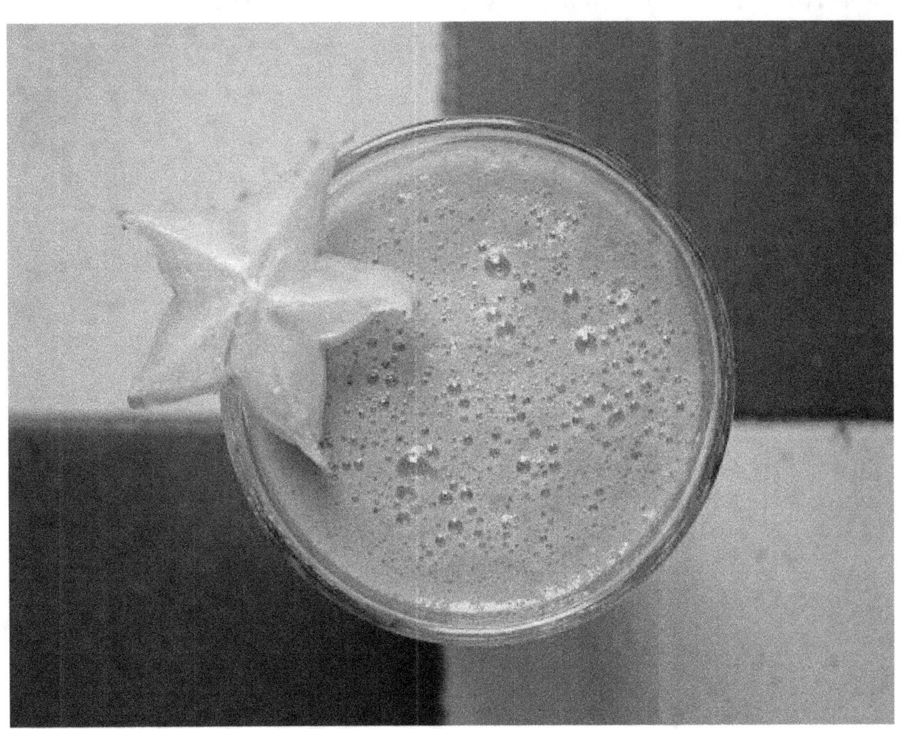

Coconut Yogurt Berry Smoothie

A dairy-free yogurt is an option if you're interested in trying coconut cultured yogurt, which contains many of the same nutrients and probiotics as the dairy version, only without any animal byproducts. This type of vegan yogurt is popular in some natural food stores and is becoming increasingly more available in regular grocery stores. The best option for smoothies is plain or vanilla, though if you want to reduce the level of sugar in your diet, then plain and unsweetened is the best option.

- 1 cup of coconut yogurt

- 1 cup of fresh or frozen berries

- ½ of a banana

- 1 teaspoon vanilla extract

- 2 cups of coconut or almond milk

- 1 tablespoon sweetener

Combine and blend the coconut yogurt and milk for 30 seconds, then add the berries, banana, vanilla extract, and sweetener, and pulse for one minute. If desired, add some ice to crush into the smoothie, then serve.

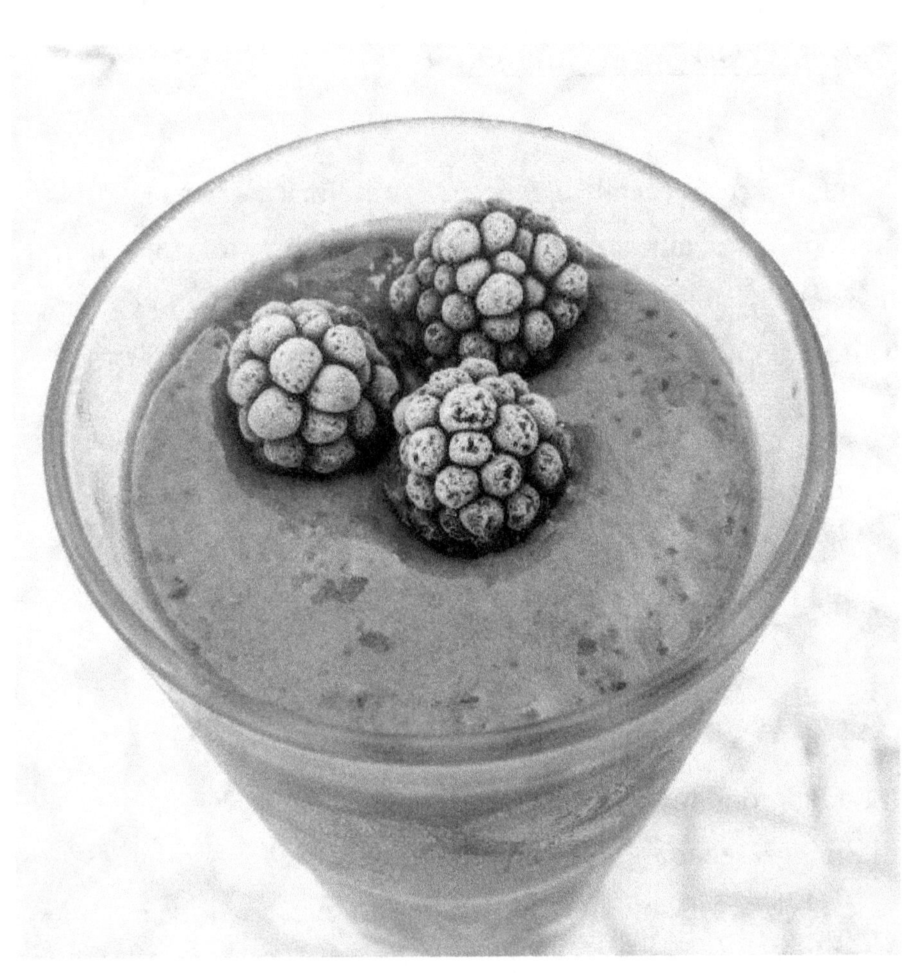

Almond Cocoa Energy Smoothie

Almonds are an excellent source of protein. This recipe blends cocoa powder, almond milk, and almond butter to create a thick, delicious treat that satisfies your hunger and nutrient needs. This smoothie is a great option for protein and energy just before the gym.

- 2 tablespoons cocoa powder

- 2 tablespoons natural sweetener

- 2 cups of almond milk

- ½ cups of almond butter

Blend almond milk and butter together for 30 seconds, then add in the sweetener and cocoa powder and pulse for another 30 seconds or until smooth. Makes two servings. Preparation time: five minutes.

There are a few variations to consider for this recipe:

- Add a banana for a thicker smoothie

- 1 teaspoon of the almond extract can be added to strengthen the almond flavor.

- Replace the almond butter with another nut-based butter, such as peanut butter, tahini, or hazelnut butter

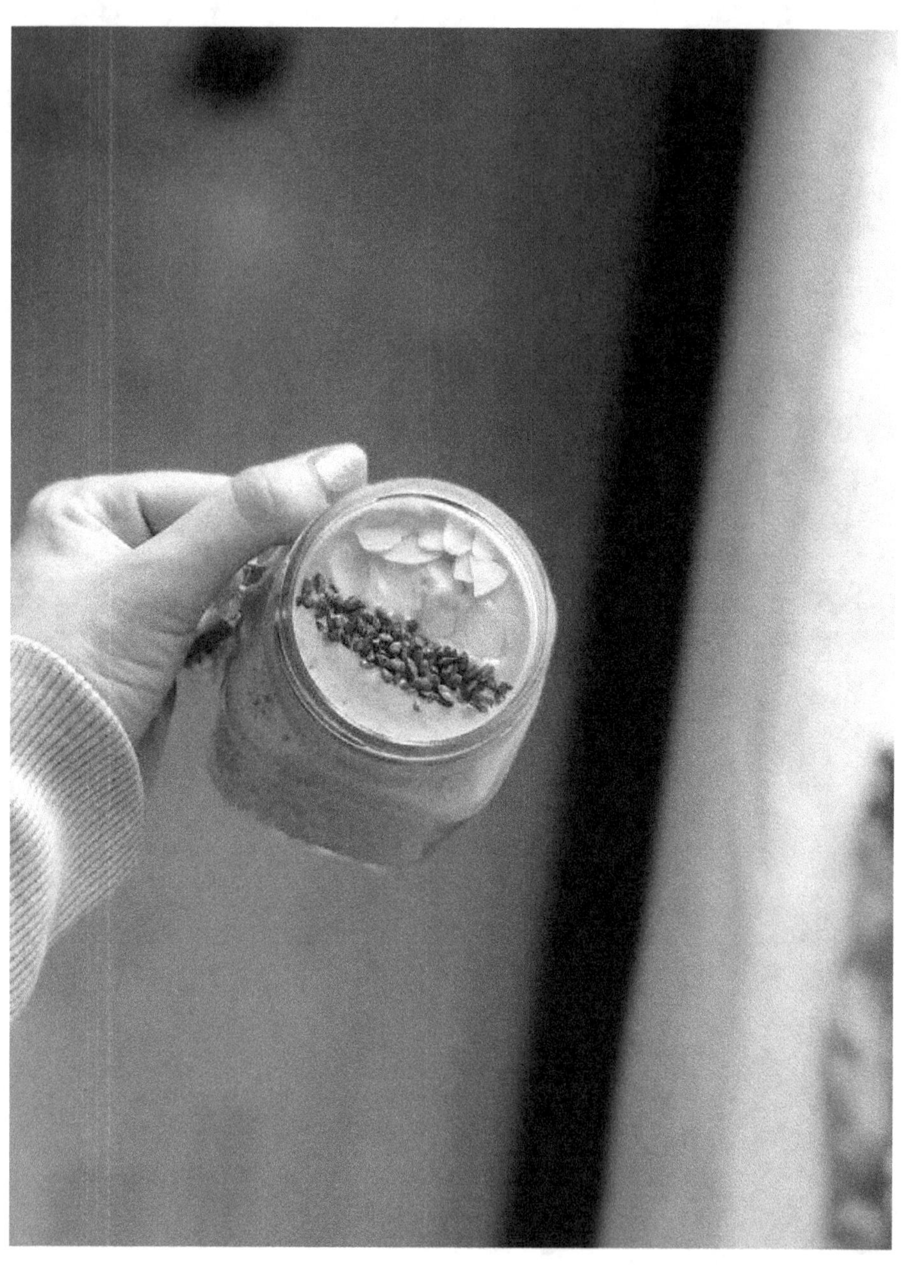

Pumpkin Cinnamon Smoothie

This smoothie is a variation on a pumpkin spice theme, by minimizing the number of spices to just cinnamon to keep it simple. If desired, pumpkin spice or the combination of cinnamon, nutmeg, and cloves can also be added for a full pumpkin spice flavor.

- ½ of a banana

- 2 teaspoons of cinnamon

- 2 teaspoons natural sweetener

- 1 cup of pumpkin puree (canned or fresh, with seeds removed)

- 2 cups of almond milk

The pumpkin puree and almond milk should be blended first in a blender until they are smoothly combined. Add the banana, sweetener, and cinnamon and process for another 30 seconds. Serves two portions and preparation time is two to five minutes.

Do you want to make this a pumpkin spice smoothie? Replace the cinnamon in this recipe with the following:

- ¼ teaspoon of cloves

- 1 teaspoon of nutmeg

- 1 teaspoon of cinnamon

Combine the three spices in a small, separate bowl, and blend with the ingredients. The banana can be substituted with an extra ½ cup of pumpkin puree.

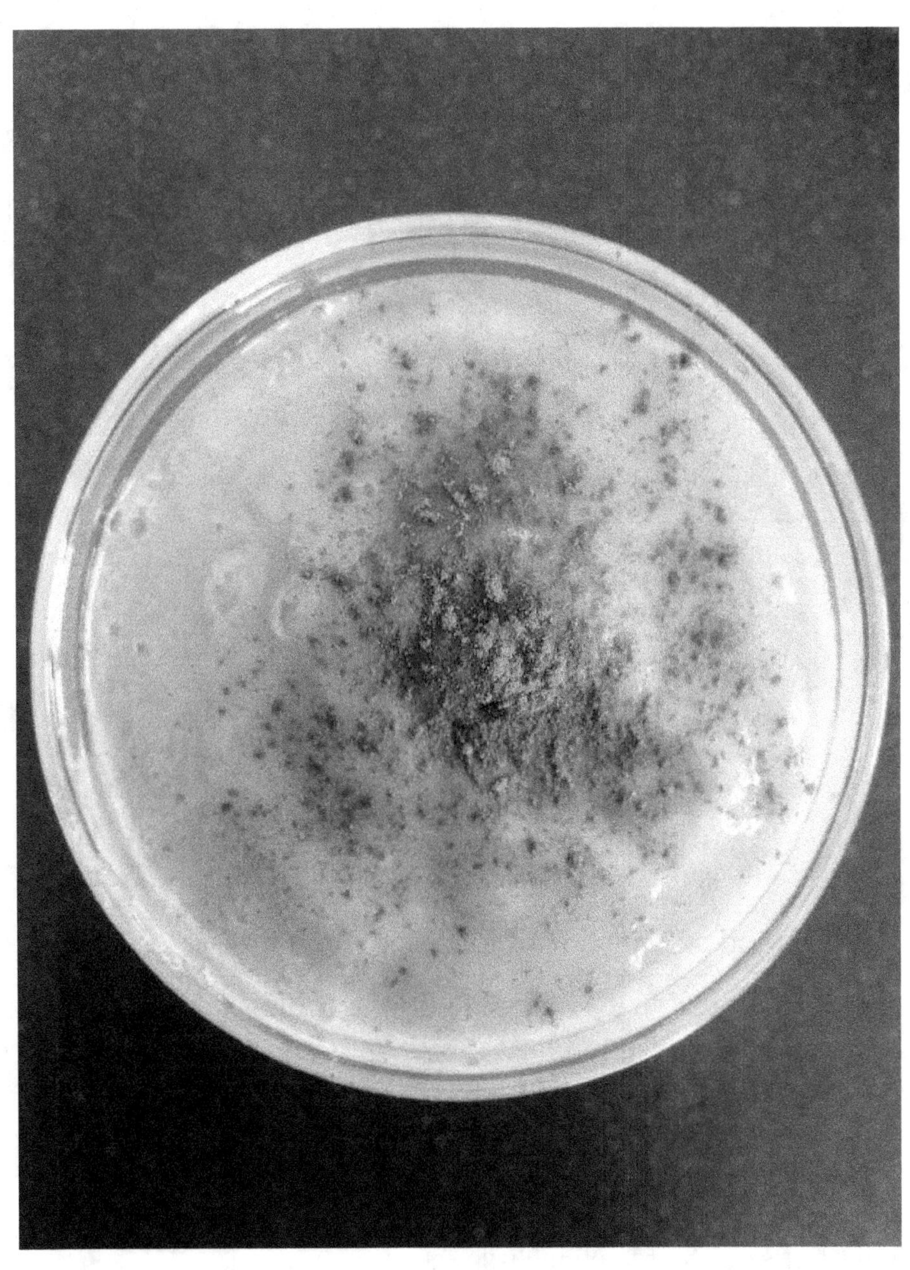

Cherries and Peaches Smoothie

Cherries are naturally sweet to taste, and a scoop of sweetener may not be needed in this smoothie. Coupled with a fresh peach, this recipe is an ideal treat at any time of the day, including breakfast. Cherries are high in alkaline, which helps with digestion and reducing pain from inflammation.

- I large ripe peach (soft), pit removed and sliced

- 1 cup of put cherries (fresh or frozen)

- 2 cups of coconut or almond milk

- 1 tablespoon of natural sweetener (optional)

- 1 teaspoon of vanilla extract (optional)

- ½ cups of crushed ice

Combine and mix the milk and cherries for 20 seconds, then add in the peach, sweetener, and vanilla, and blend again, then add in the ice. This smoothie serves two and takes five minutes to prepare.

Variations on the recipe include the following:

- Replace the peach with a ripe mango

- Instead of cherries, use 1 cup of raspberries

- Add a banana to thicken the drink

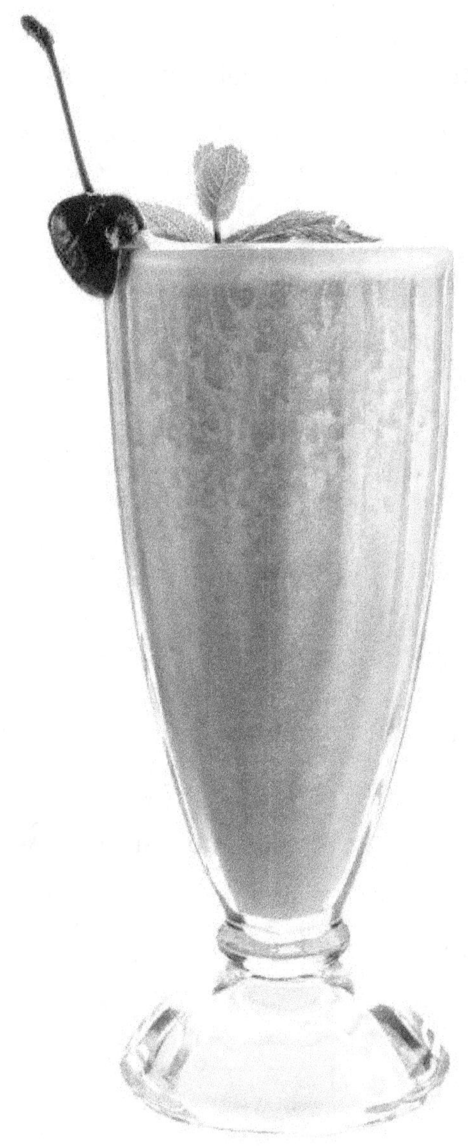

Mango Pistachio Smoothie

Mangoes are sweet and make an excellent ingredient for smoothies for this reason. Their flavor works well with a variety of other fruits, such as pineapple, coconut, papaya, and banana. Pistachios are added to boost this smoothie with a dose of protein.

- ¼ cups if crushed pistachios

- 2 cups of coconut milk

- ½ cups of coconut yogurt

- 2 medium mangoes, pits removed and sliced

- 2 teaspoons of natural sweetener

- ½ of a banana (optional)

Blend the milk, yogurt, and mangoes together and blend for 20 seconds. Add in the sweetener, banana (optional) and pistachios and continue to mix. If needed, add more milk if the smoothie becomes too thick. Top with pistachios before serving. This recipe makes two servings and the preparation time is five minutes.

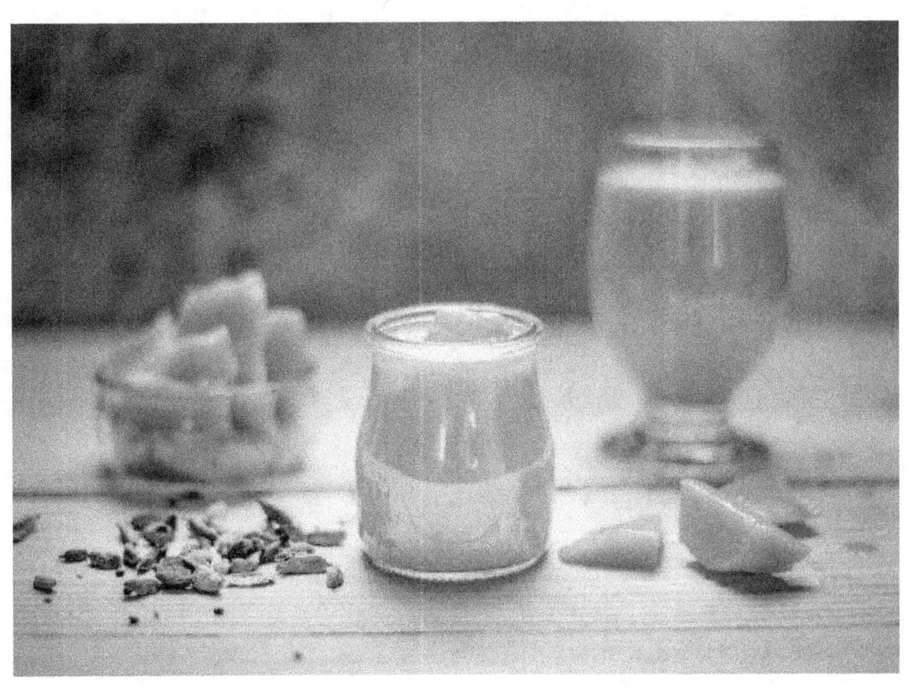

**Kiwi, Strawberry, and Banana Smoothie**

The sweetness of strawberries combined with the sour taste of kiwis creates a tasty blend with a banana and milk. Blackberries, raspberries, or blueberries can be added or used in place of the strawberries when they are not available.

- 1 cup of strawberries (sliced and stems removed)

- 1 kiwi, sliced and peeled

- 2 tablespoons of sweetener

- 2 cups of almond milk

- 1 banana

Combine the milk, banana, and berries in the blender and mix. Then, add in the kiwi and sweetener and blend for another 20 seconds, until smooth, then serve. This recipe makes two servings and takes 6-8 minutes to prepare.

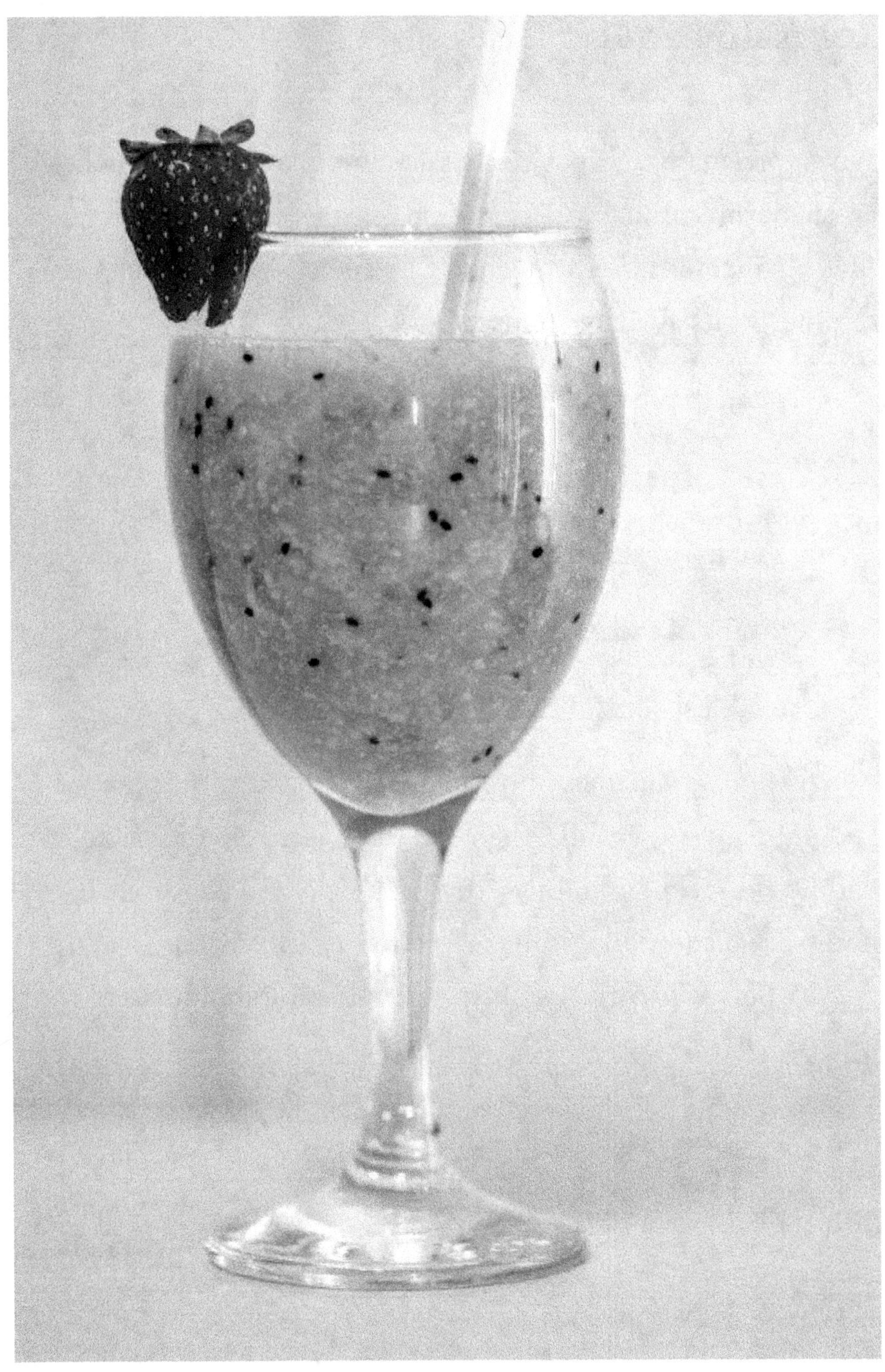

**Tropical Smoothie**

Pineapple, mango, papaya, and coconut milk are combined to create a tropical-inspired smoothie. This is a tasty, rich treat that can include other tropical fruits, such as guava and banana, or other fruits available to use.

- 1 cup of pineapple, sliced

- 1 cup of papaya, sliced

- ½ cups of sliced mangoes

- 2 cups of coconut milk

- 2 tablespoons of sweetener

Add the milk, mangoes, pineapple, and papaya to the blender and pulse for 30 seconds, then add the sweetener and pulse for another 10 seconds, adding extra milk if needed (this may be necessary if additional fruits are added, such as bananas and/or guava). Serves two and can be prepared in 6-8 minutes.

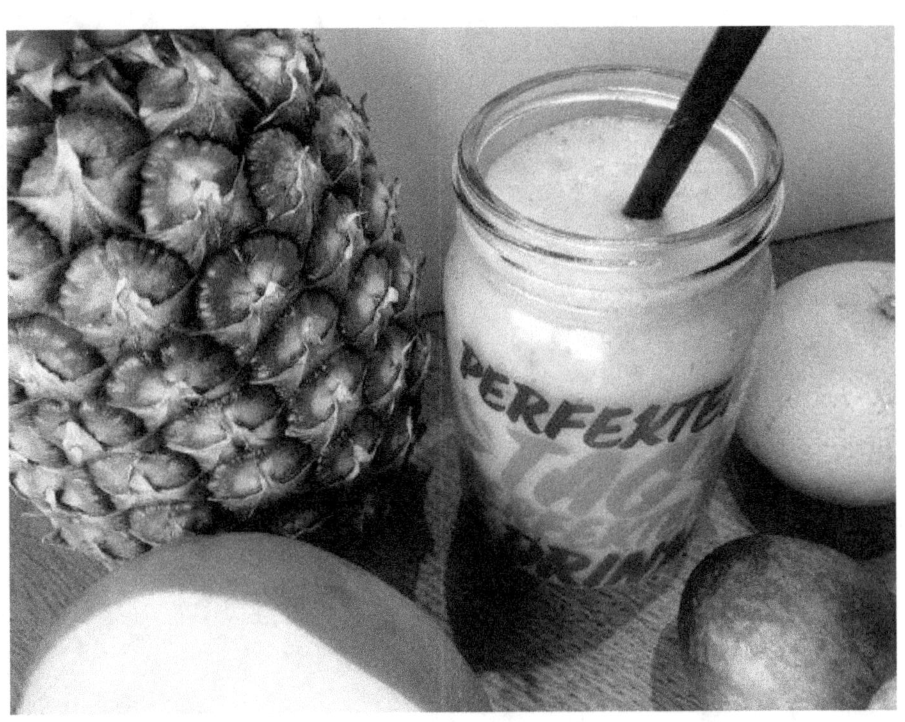

Peanut Butter Smoothie

The ultimate protein smoothie, peanut butter is high in healthy fats and protein, and can easily be added to create a delicious smoothie. There is the option of adding cocoa powder for additional flavor, though this recipe is tasty just with the peanut butter on its own, or with a banana. Choose peanut butter with little or no salt, and without sugar, as you can add your own type of sweetener as desired. Almond or hemp milk can be added to boost the protein content, especially if you're embarking on a long jog or bicycle ride.

- 2 cups of almond or hemp milk

- 1 cup of peanut butter

- 2 tablespoons of sweetener

- 1 banana

- ¼ cups of crushed peanuts

Combine the milk, peanut butter, and sweetener into the blender and mix for 30 seconds or until smooth. Add in the banana and crushed peanuts to blend for another 20 seconds, then serve. This smoothie makes two servings and can be prepared in under six minutes.

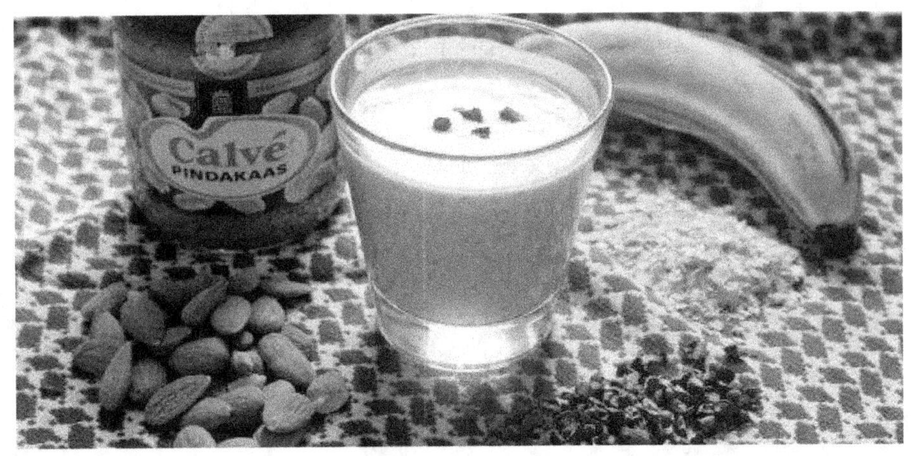

Calvé
PINDAKAAS

Tahini and Maple Syrup Smoothie

This is one of the only smoothies that does not contain fruit, though it is a decadent treat that combines the nutty flavor of tahini with the sweetness of maple syrup. A banana can be added to boost the fiber content of this recipe.

- 1 ½ cups of almond milk

- ¾ cups of tahini

- 2 tablespoons of maple syrup

- 1 banana (optional)

Combine and mix in a blender the tahini, milk, and maple syrup for a quarter of a minute. Add in the banana (if desired), extra milk as needed, and process for another 20 seconds, then serve. This recipe makes about two servings and takes about five minutes to prepare.

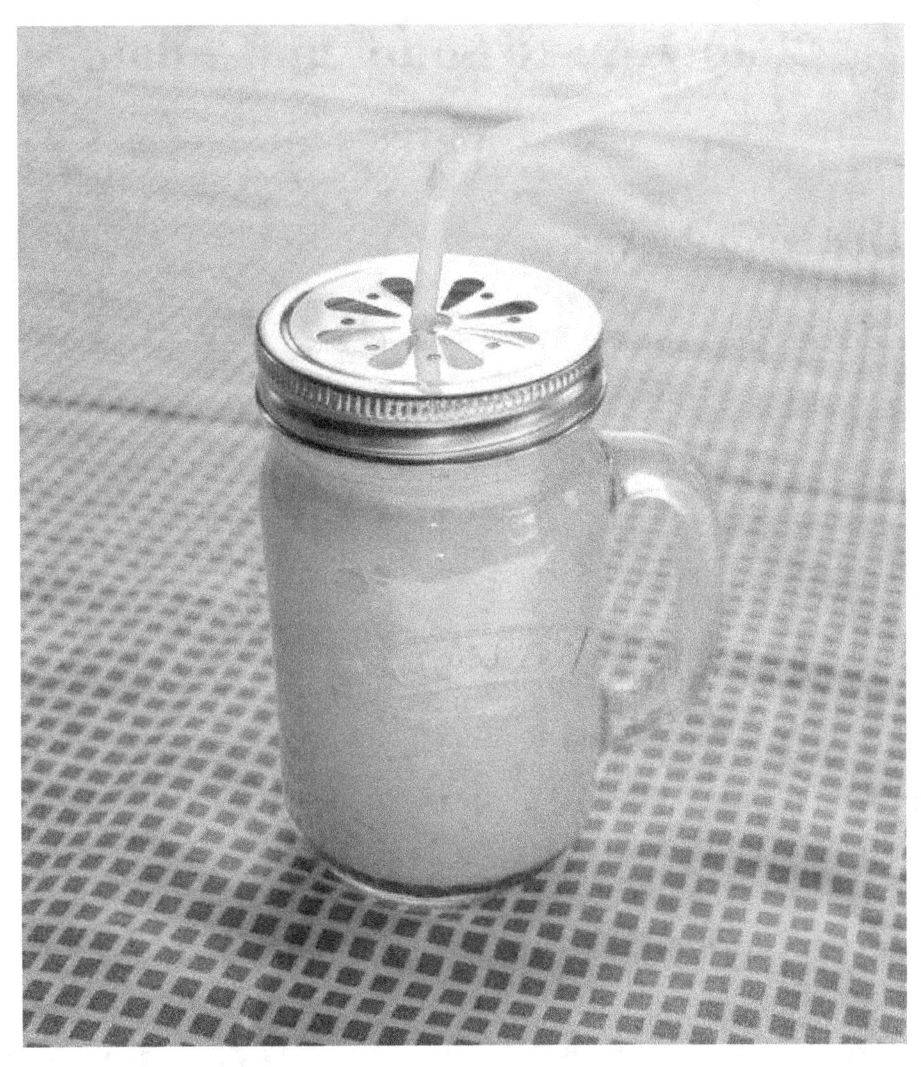

Chapter 4: 10 Soups and Salad Recipes

Five Soup Recipes

<u>*Miso Soup*</u>

A popular soup in Asian cuisine, miso soup is tasty, easy to make, and healthy. Most grocery stores and natural or specialty food stores offer dried miso in soup-making kits or as a paste that can be added to soups and sauces. Miso is available in white, yellow, and red varieties, where the white is mild in flavor (fermented over several weeks or on month), yellow is slightly stronger (several months of fermenting), and red is the strongest, most pungent flavor (several months or more – up to one year of fermentation). White and yellow are most commonly used, as their flavors are mild and easy to combine with other ingredients.

- 2-3 tablespoons miso paste

- 3-4 cups of water

- ½ cup of mushroom, sliced

- 1 cup of green onion, chopped

- 1 cup of sliced tofu (small cubes, ½-inch each)

- 1 cup of dried seaweed (nori)

In a small cooking pot, boil the water and add in the miso paste, stirring consistently for ten minutes or longer, until boiling. Add in the tofu, seaweed, and mushrooms, and continue cooking until all ingredients are tender. Serve and toss in the green onions. This soup is often served with sushi or sashimi and can also be paired with stir-fries or roasts.

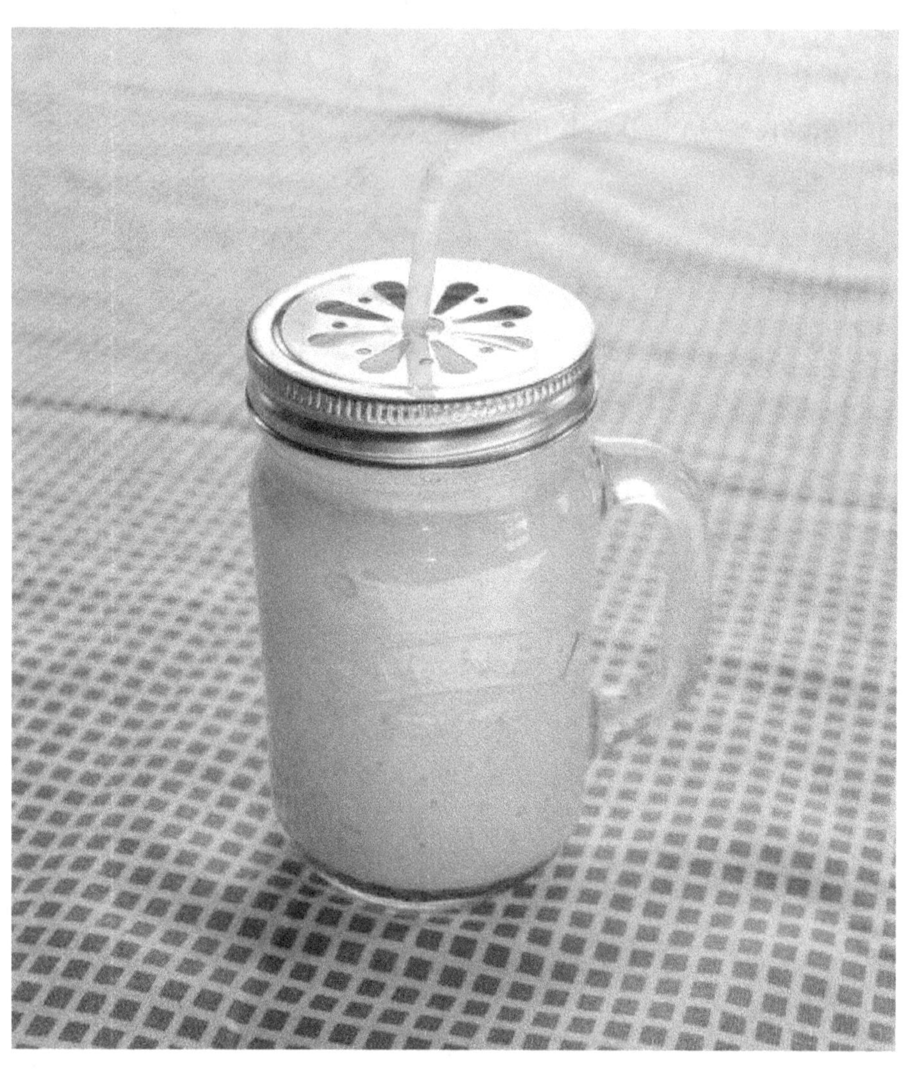

Vegetable Broth

Creating a tasty, nutritious vegetable broth is the basis for creating many delicious soups and stews. The vegan broth is readily available in most grocery stores, though it is ideal to make it from scratch, which allows you to customize the ingredients you include based on your preferences. For example, you may want to add more onion and garlic than a standard broth, as well as certain herbs and spices. Preparing a broth can take up to twenty hours to fully saturate the flavor of the vegetable into the water so that it can be strong enough to provide a base to many other soups.

To get started, choose the vegetables you want, and include peelings, peels, and leftovers from other meals to reduce the amount of waste:

- Onions, including skins

- Garlic cloves and leftover skins and feelings

- Shredded cabbage, stems, etc.

- Kale and other leafy greens (include the stems)

- Carrots

- Celery

- Bay leaves

- Dried herbs, leaves, and spices (sage, basil, etc.)

- Potato peels and skins

- Yam peels and skins

- Dried chili pepper

Pour 6-8 cups of water in a large cooking pot. The amount of water can be adjusted according to the number of vegetables and other ingredients included to ensure they are adequately covered. Add in all the ingredients (above) or a similar assortment according to preference and bring to a boil. Add sea salt and any additional spices or flavors and continue boiling for 15-20 mins. Lower the fire in the stove and gently boil for another 5-6 hours. If you need to turn off the stove, leave the pot covered and reheat later. It can take up to 20 hours to adequately transfer all the flavors to the water to make the soup base or broth. Once this is done, drain and use the broth to make other soups, or enjoy in a small bowl or cup. It will last for about a week if the broth is stored in a fridge. It will last up to 3 months if stored in the freezer.

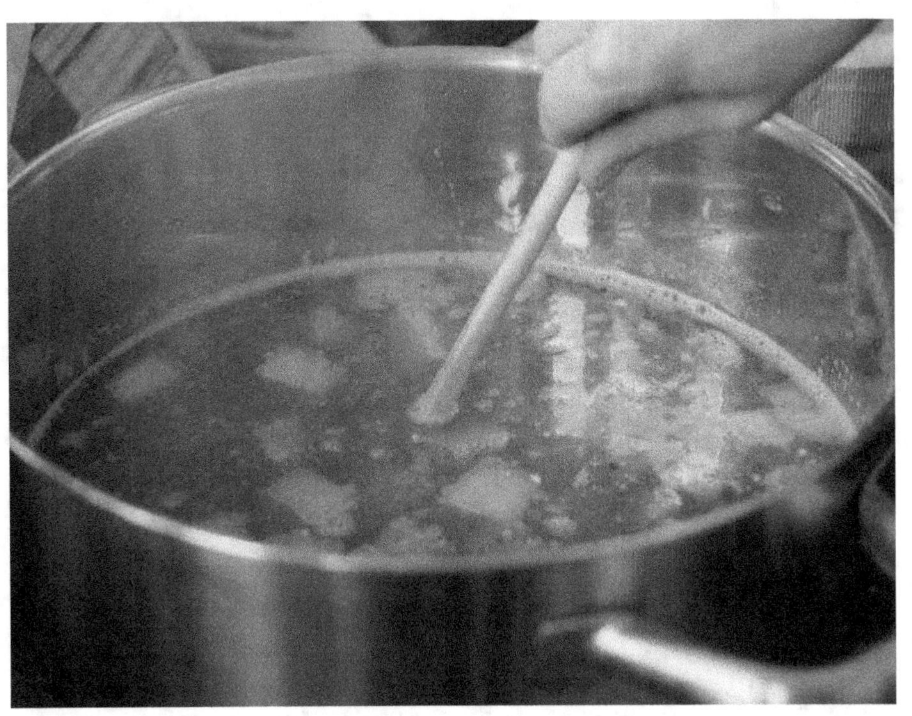

Butternut Squash Soup

This is a tasty soup that's mild and pleasant in flavor. Butternut squash is the variety used for this recipe, though any type of squash can be used if available. To prepare the squash, bake in the oven for 30 minutes whole at 375 degrees, and poke several holes with a fork to allow the inside to cook well. After 30 minutes, remove from the oven, slice in half or quarters, and bake again in almost half an hour in the same baking sheet that has been lined with parchment paper. Remove the seeds and scoop the flesh of the squash into a bowl, then set aside.

- 1 butternut squash, roasted, seeded, and flesh removed

- 4 cups of vegetable broth

- ½ cup of chopped onion

- 2 teaspoons of thyme

- 1 cup of coconut milk

- 1 teaspoon of black pepper

Bring the four cups of vegetable broth to a boil, then add in the onion, baked squash, thyme, black pepper, and coconut milk. Lower the heat and cook on medium, stirring regularly for another 15-20 minutes. Remove from the stove to cool, and process until smooth in the blender in batches. Pour the soup again in the same pot so that it can be reheated, then add more thyme, black pepper, and serve. This recipe makes approximately 4-6 servings and can take 1.5 hours to prepare (including roasting the squash).

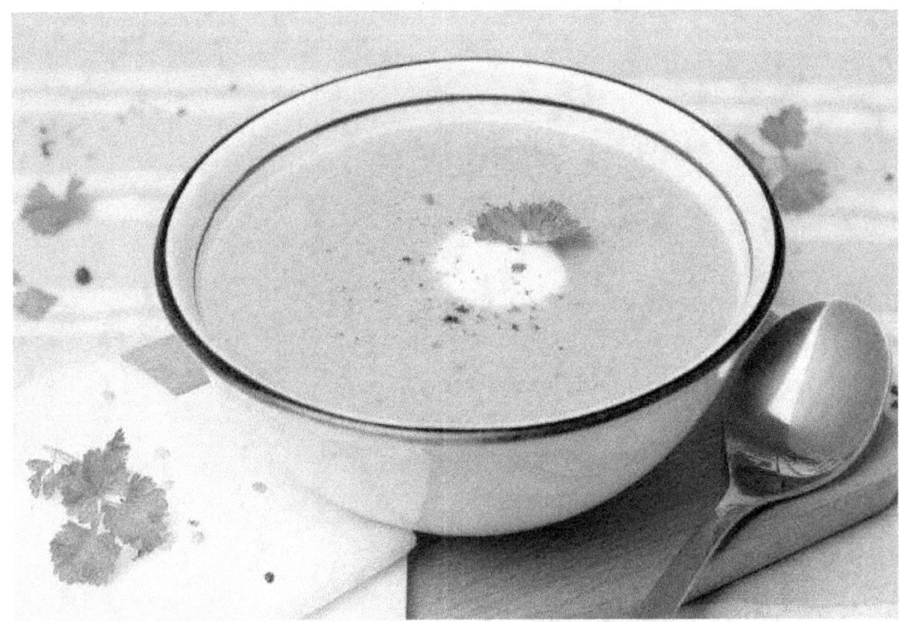

Ginger Carrot Soup

This is a tasty soup that combines the mellow, sweet taste of carrots with the strong impression of ginger for a warming soup. This recipe uses 5 cups of vegetable broth and 3 cups of sliced carrots, which may require extra preparation time to slice the carrots and make the broth unless it is store-bought.

- 2 diced onions

- 5 cups of vegetable broth

- 3-4 cups of carrots, sliced

- 2 teaspoons of ground ginger (fresh)

- 1 teaspoon of black pepper

- Dried or fresh parsley, for garnish

- 1 cup of coconut milk

- ½ cup of vegan sour cream

Cook the onions, carrots, and olive oil in a cooking pot that is large in size for about eight minutes in medium-heat setting, or until soft.

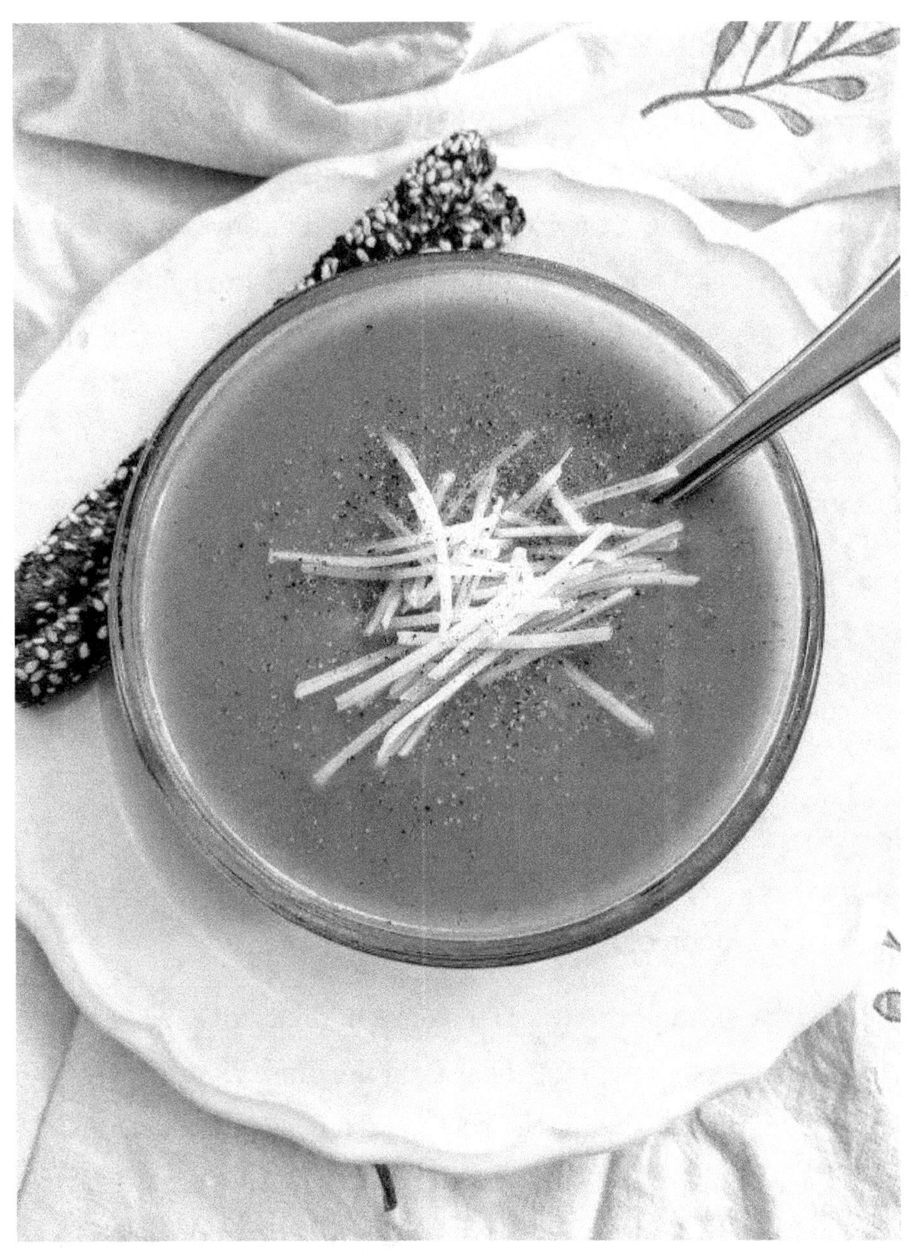

Green Pea Soup

A slightly sweet and savory dish, green pea soup is easy to prepare and makes a tasty dish in a vegan diet. Frozen or fresh peas can be used and are recommended due to their flavor (canned peas are another option, though they don't taste quite the same).

- 1 bag of frozen peas

- 2 tablespoons of olive oil

- 1 onion, chopped

- 3 cups of vegetable broth

- 1 teaspoon of dill (fresh or dried)

- 1 teaspoon of tarragon

- 1 teaspoon of black pepper

Use a large-sized pot to warm the olive oil in a stove temperature set in medium-heat. Add the onion, simmering for a couple of minutes. Pour the broth and spices (tarragon, dill, and black pepper) and continue to cook, then increase the heat so that it begins to boil. Lower the heat and add in the peas and cook on low-medium for about 10-15 minutes until peas are tender, then remove and chill. Use a food processor to pulse the soup batch by batch. Serve hot or cold. This recipe makes 4-6 servings and takes about 30 minutes.

Add a dollop of coconut yogurt or sour cream on top of the soup when serving.

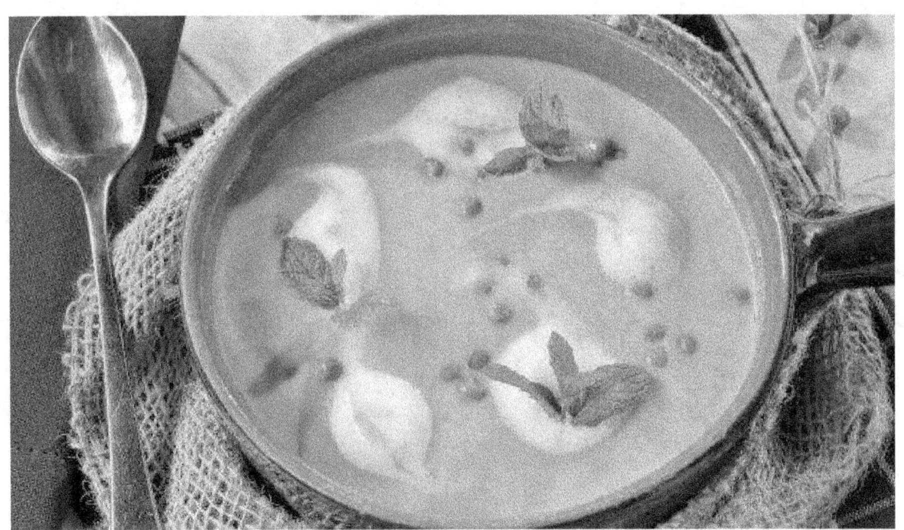

Five Salad Recipes

Salads don't have to be the boring side dishes most people consider them to be or the small handful of leaves next to the main course. Salads can be the dinner or side dish and with much more flavor and excitement than their traditional variations. Each of these recipes combines a few or more tastes that contrast and compliment at once. These are great for lunch, for a meal on-the-go, or a potluck.

Quinoa Salad

This salad is a full meal on its own, as it contains all the nutrients you need in just one serving. Quinoa makes an excellent base with a variety of fresh vegetables, herbs, nuts, and seeds.

- 1 cup of uncooked quinoa

- 1 small or medium cucumber (sliced, about one cup)

- 2 cups of water

- 2 cups of bok choy

- 1 red bell pepper, diced

- ½ cup of dried cranberries and/or blueberries

- ½ cups of mixed sunflower seeds, pumpkin seeds, crushed walnuts, pecans, and other nuts

- ½ cups of fresh parsley, dill, mint, basil, and/or cilantro

For the dressing:

- Dash of sea salt

- 1 teaspoon of maple syrup or low carb sweetener

- 2 tablespoons of apple cider vinegar

- 3 tablespoons of olive oil

- Dash of black pepper

- 2 tablespoons of lemon juice (freshly squeezed)

In preparing the dressing, you need to put together first and mix all the ingredients for the dressing in a small mixing container before setting it aside. Combine the salad ingredients and toss evenly, then serve with the vinaigrette. This dish makes about 4-6 servings and takes about 15-20 minutes to prepare.

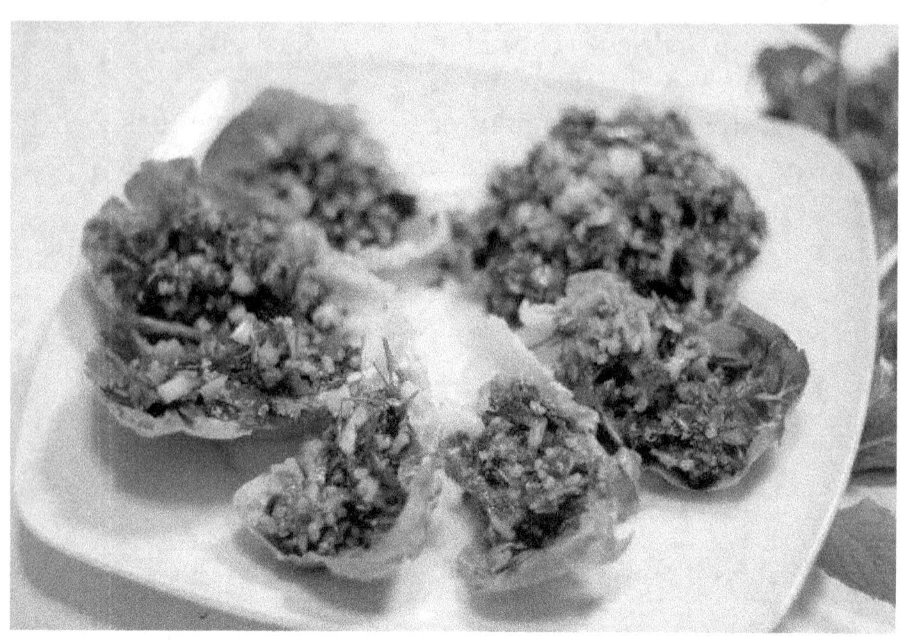

Kale Blueberry Salad

Kale is a superfood that contains a healthy dose of calcium, protein, fiber, and antioxidants. It's a bitter-tasting vegetable that compliments a wide range of flavors, sweet, spicy, and savory. This salad gives kale a lift with a sweet infusion of blueberries and a three-ingredient vinaigrette.

- 1 cup of fresh blueberries

- ½ cups of sliced almonds

- 1 bunch of kale (stems removed, sliced or shredded)

For the dressing:

- 1 teaspoon of maple syrup

- 2 tablespoons of lime or lemon juice

- 2 teaspoons of olive oil

Mix the three ingredients for the vinaigrette in a mixing dish that is small in size before setting it aside. In a larger bowl, combine the sliced kale, and toss in the fresh blueberries. Serve sprinkled with the vinaigrette and topped with sliced almonds.

There are a few variations to consider for this salad:

- Lightly toast the almond slices in a skillet for one minute before topping

- Use 1 teaspoon of blueberry marmalade instead of maple syrup for the dressing

Note: There are many types of kale to choose from (red, curly, black kale) and all or any if they are suitable for this salad.

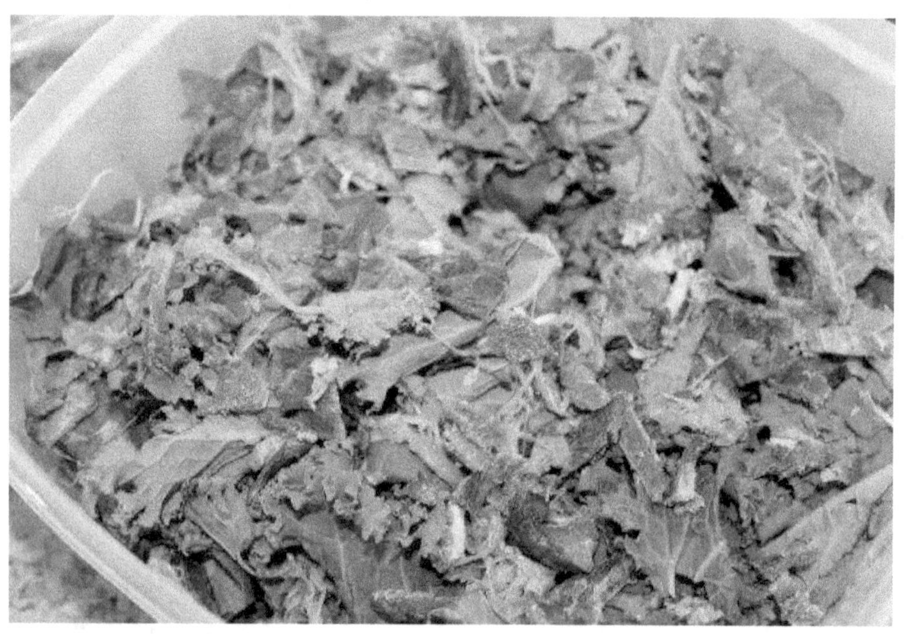

Spinach, Mandarin, and Walnut Salad

Spinach is an excellent source of iron and calcium. Combined with mandarin and walnuts, there's a good source of vitamins and fiber as well. The dressing used for this salad adds a citrus flavor and maple syrup.

- 1 bunch of spinach, washed and drained

- 3-4 mandarins, peeled and pieces (slices) removed

- 1 cup of coarsely chopped walnuts

- ½ cup of shredded carrots

For the dressing:

- 2 teaspoons of olive oil

- 3 teaspoons of orange juice (freshly squeezed)

- 1 teaspoon of maple syrup

Mix the ingredients for the salad dressing in a small bowl and set aside. In a larger bowl, add the fresh spinach (washed and drained in a colander), and toss in the shredded carrots, walnuts, and mandarin slices. Serve with dressing. This recipe makes approximately 4-5 servings and can be prepared within 15 minutes.

**Arugula and Roasted Pear Salad**

This recipe features a roasted pear, which adds a naturally mellow and sweet flavor to the arugula and other ingredients. Pecans and walnuts are added to balance the texture and flavors. Crumbled vegan cheese can also be added as a topping, if available.

- ½ cups chopped walnuts

- 1 cup of coarsely chopped pecans

- 2 cups of chopped arugula

- 1 roasted pear, sliced in half

For the dressing:

- 1 teaspoon of maple syrup

- 2 teaspoons of lime juice

- 2 teaspoons of olive oil

To roast the pear, set the oven to 350, slice the pear in half, and place face down on a baking sheet prepared with a parchment paper. Bake for half an hour, then remove and cool for 10-15 minutes. Mix the dressing ingredients together well, then set aside. Combine all the salad items and blend evenly. Lightly coat with dressing and serve.

Options for this salad include the following:

- Add ½ cup of dried cranberries

- Sliced coconut chips (approx. ¼ cup)

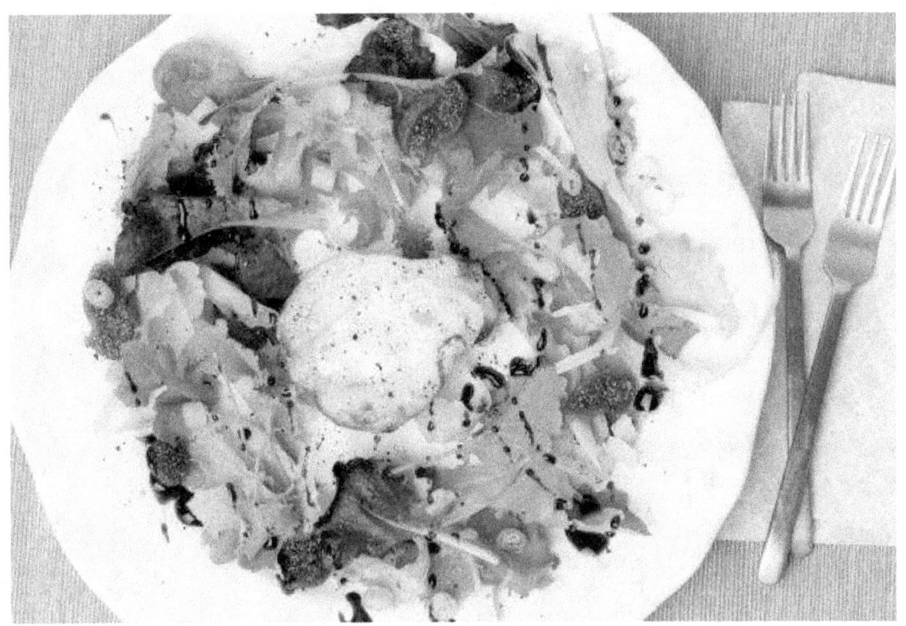

Fruit Salad

This is-a fun and effortless salad to prepare, which includes adding and combining the fruit options of your choice. When selecting fruits, make sure they are fresh and in season. Frozen fruit can be used, though it would need to thaw first, and may not have the same texture (berries are the best option if frozen fruit is used). The list below is a suggested combination of fruits to include in this recipe:

- 1 large apple, sliced (skin can be removed or left on)
- 1-2 mandarins, peeled and broken apart into slices/pieces or one large orange, sliced and skin removed
- 1 cup of grapes (seedless)
- 1 cup of sliced cantaloupe or honeydew into cubes
- 1 cup of sliced watermelon
- ½ cup of sliced strawberries stems removed
- ½ cup of blueberries
- ½ cup of raspberries
- 1 cup of sliced pineapples

This salad is easy to prepare and may include as little or as many of the fruits above (and more). Wash, chop, and assemble all fruits and drain in a colander. Serve with freshly squeezed lemon and garnish with fresh mint leaves. The salad serves 4-6 and takes approximately 15-20 minutes to prepare.

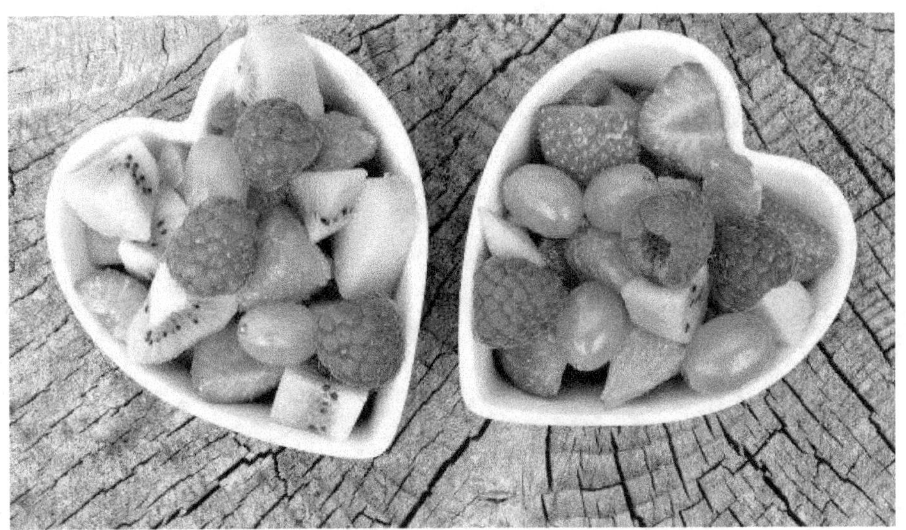

Chapter 5: 10 Main Dish Recipes

Main Meal Recipes and Sides

There are many options for vegan dinners, both the main feature and the side dishes. Tofu and tempeh often play a central role in main dishes, though many pulses and vegetables, including grains, can take center stage as well. The following recipes focus on several options that can be varied, whether your focus is tofu or tempeh, beans, or a wide range of vegetables in one dish.

Lentil Dal

One of the most popular Indian dishes, lentil dal is an excellent choice for many reasons: it's high in fiber, protein, and calcium. Turmeric, a spice used in this recipe, contains high amounts of antioxidants and fights inflammation in the body. This dish can be prepared mild, or with some added spice. Any lentils can be used, though red lentils are best, as they cook easily and mix well with the other ingredients.

- 1 green chili pepper, diced (with stem removed)
- 1 cup of diced onion (white or yellow)

- 1 tablespoon of olive oil

- 2 teaspoons of cumin seeds

- 1 cup of red lentils

- 1 teaspoon of cinnamon

- 4 crushed garlic cloves

- 2 teaspoons of grated ginger (fresh is recommended)

- 1 small or medium tomato, diced

- 1 teaspoon of paprika

- ½ teaspoon of cardamom

- 1 teaspoon of turmeric

- 1 teaspoon of sea salt

- 1 teaspoon of lemon juice

- 1 teaspoon of chili powder (optional)

- 1 cup of chopped parsley or cilantro leaves

If using dried lentils, rinse and bring to a boil in a saucepan covered in water, reduce, and cook on medium for 15-20 minutes. While the lentils are cooking, let a skillet heat up before adding the olive oil, cumin, and cinnamon on medium for five minutes, then add in the garlic, onion, green chili, chili powder (optional ingredient), and ginger. Simmer for another five or six minutes, then add the following items: salt, tomatoes, paprika, cardamom, and turmeric. Continue to cook for another five minutes. When the lentils are cooked, drain and stir in the skillet mixed with the lentils, combining evenly. Add fresh lemon juice. Serve with cilantro or parsley leaves.

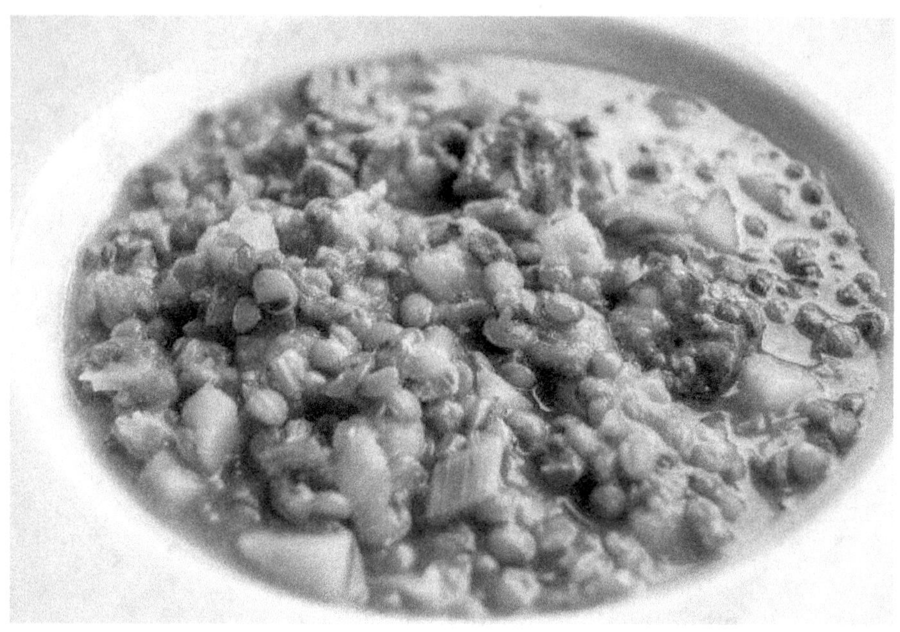

Tofu Bake with Squash

This recipe is basically two sides in one to create a nourishing meal. Squash bakes well alongside tofu, and both are done within the same time frame, which makes this an easy meal to prepare. The only additional preparation for the tofu involves marinating in the following three ingredients:

- ½ cup of olive oil

- 1 cup of soy sauce (use low sodium, if you require less salt in your diet)

- 2 teaspoons of sesame oil (optional)

- 2 tablespoons of lemon juice

Combine all the above ingredients in a bowl and set aside. Rinse and drain one package (or block) of firm tofu and set aside in a small or medium food keeper. The tofu should be covered with the marinade. Place in the refrigerate for two hours at a minimum. When the tofu is ready, drain and retain ½ cups of the liquid and set aside. Heat in an oven to 350. In a baking dish of medium size, lay the marinated tofu and place two halves of a squash beside the tofu (if there isn't enough room, use two baking dishes; one for the tofu and one for the squash.) Pour the ½ cup of retained liquid from the marinade over the tofu, and if desired, coat in sesame seeds. Bake with the squash for 35-45 minutes, until the tofu is slightly crispy, and the squash is tender inside.

This dish makes about 4-6 servings and works well with a dark leafy green salad or cooked spinach. A small bowl of miso soup makes an excellent side, or a slightly thicker version of a miso-based soup can be poured over the squash before serving.

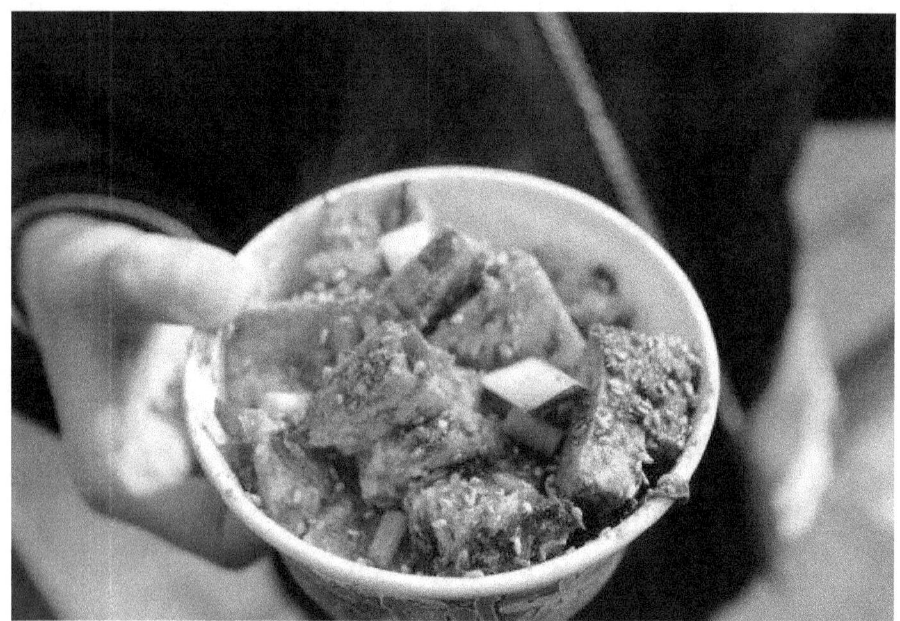

Sweet and Sour Tempeh Skillet

Tempeh is fermented soy food which a strong, textured taste similar to meat. Like tofu, tempeh takes on the flavors of other foods it is cooked with, and marinating is one of the best methods of getting the most out of tempeh. In this recipe, a sweet and sour marinade is prepared by combining the following ingredients and covering one block of tempeh (sliced into cubes) and refrigerated for two hours:

- 3 tablespoons of olive oil

- ½ cup of orange or pineapple juice

- 1 teaspoon of maple syrup

- 3 teaspoons of vinegar (white wine vinegar)

- 2 teaspoons soy sauce

Mix these ingredients thoroughly in a small bowl, then cover the tempeh in a sealed container and chill for a minimum of two hours.

The skillet meal consists of the following ingredients:

- ½ cup of pineapple, cut into small cubes

- 1 clove of garlic, diced

- 1 red onion, diced

- 1 block of marinated tempeh (as shown above)

- ½ cup of snow peas

- ½ cup of chopped celery

- ½ cup of sliced carrots

- 1 or 2 bell peppers, sliced

- 2 teaspoons ground ginger

- 2 teaspoons of soy sauce

- 2 tablespoons of olive oil

Heat the skillet on medium heat with olive oil. Add and sauté the onion and garlic. Continue cooking it for a couple of minutes. In the meantime, remove the tempeh and drain, retaining ½ cup of the liquid. Add the tempeh and liquid to the skillet and cook for ten mins, then add in the rest of the ingredients before continuing to gently boil on low or medium for another 10-15 minutes, until the vegetables are cooked but still crispy. Remove from heat and serve with rice or noodles.

Some variations to consider for this recipe include the following:

- Sprinkle with raw or lightly toasted sesame seeds

- Add a couple of teaspoons of crushed peanuts as a topping

- Serve with fresh sliced pineapple instead of or in addition to the cooked version included in this recipe.

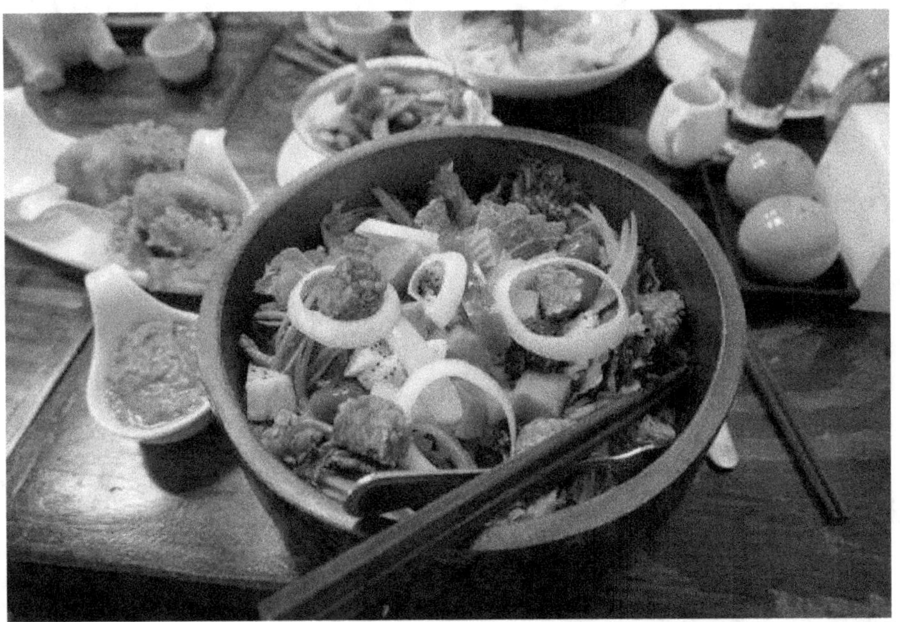

Veggie Skillet Dinner

This dish is full of nutrients, including dome leafy greens to increase your intake of iron and calcium. If you want to explore a wide variety of textures, flavors, and combinations, this is an opportunity to mix a lot of options together. For this dish, it's advantageous to use a large wok or similarly sized skillet to contain a large volume of vegetables. Consider adding all or some of the following:

Vegetables:

- Snow peas
- Carrots
- Celery
- Bok choy
- Broccoli
- Cauliflower
- Bell peppers
- Green chilies
- Bean sprouts

- Mushrooms (any variety – shitake, Portobello, or button mushrooms)

- Baby corn

- Onions (white, red, or yellow)

- Garlic

- Chopped raw spinach

- Kale leaves, chopped

Herbs and leaves:

- Basil leaves

- Parsley

- Tarragon

- Bay leaves

- Curry spice or leaves

Other ingredients:

- Soy sauce

- Teriyaki sauce

- Sesame seeds

- Sliced almonds

- Mandarin slices or pineapple chunks

Heat the wok or large skillet on medium and add olive oil, followed by teriyaki or soy sauce (chili or curry paste are also options), then add the desired herbs and spices and continue to simmer. Add in the vegetables that take the longest to cook first: celery, carrots, broccoli, cauliflower, etc. and cook for 10-15 minutes before adding the remaining ingredients, leaving the mushrooms and bean sprouts last, as they fry quickly. Sprinkle with nuts and/or leaves. Serve with mandarin or pineapple chunks, if preferred, or add them in while cooking (or omit completely).

There are some interesting variations: add tamarind for a Phad Thai-style flavor and serve with noodles or mix the soy sauce and olive oil with 1-2 tablespoons of peanut butter for a thicker sauce for the stir fry.

Chickpea Curry

A warm, aromatic dish, chickpea curry is an excellent meal that can be enjoyed alone, or with a small, simple side such as a salad or soup. This dish is prepared with coconut milk, which is often used as a base for curries, as it enhances the flavor and works well with garlic, onions, chili as well as a variety of species and ingredients.

- 1 large can or 1 ½ small cans of chickpeas, drained and rinsed
- 1 medium or large red onion, sliced
- 4 crushed cloves of garlic
- 2 tablespoons of grated ginger (fresh)
- 1 tablespoon of garam masala
- 1 teaspoon of black pepper
- 1 teaspoon of turmeric
- 1 large can of coconut milk, or 2 cups
- 2 cups of diced tomatoes
- 1 teaspoon of sea salt
- ½ teaspoon of cayenne pepper or chili powder

- 1 tablespoon of lemon or lime juice

- 1 cup of sliced cilantro leaves

- 2 tablespoons of olive oil

In a medium-sized skillet, let the olive oil heated before adding the garlic, salt, and red onion. Cook for a few minutes, then add in the ginger and cook another two minutes. Mix in the turmeric, black pepper, garam masala, cayenne pepper or chili powder, and tomatoes. Simmer for another 5-10 minutes, then gently pour in the coconut milk before lowering the heat. Cook on medium-low and stir continuously until coconut milk and all ingredients are done. Test taste and season with additional flavors if needed, before serving. This dish serves up to 6 people and can be served with basmati rice or rice noodles.

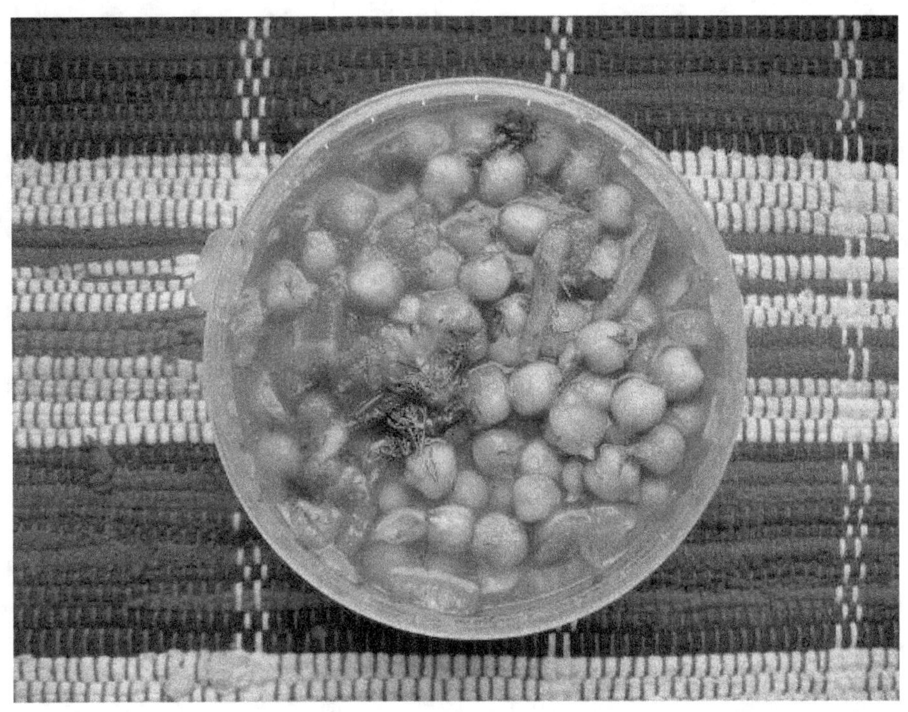

Vegan Chili

During the colder months, chili is a hearty and filling meal that is inexpensive to prepare and easy to make. There are some options to explore with this meal, including the types of beans, spices, and vegetables to include. For added protein, TVP (textured vegetable protein) can be added. This is a supplement available in dried form, found in natural food or bulk stores. It is used as a quick and effortless way to add a quick dose of protein to soups, stews, and other recipes for vegan meals.

- 2 large cans or 4-5 cups of diced tomatoes (or the same portion of fresh, sliced tomatoes)

- 1 ½ cups of tomato paste

- 4 crushed cloves of garlic

- 1 sliced onion (medium)

- 1 can of kidney beans (white or red)

- 1 can of chickpeas

- 1 can of black beans

- 1 can of pinto beans

- 1 cup of sliced carrots

- 1 cup of diced celery

- ½ cup of sliced mushrooms

- 3-4 tablespoons of chili powder

- 2 teaspoons of black pepper

- 2 jalapeno peppers, sliced

- 1 teaspoon of sea salt

- 1 tablespoon ground cumin

- 1 cup of fresh cilantro or parsley, chopped

- 2 tablespoons of textured vegetable protein (optional, only use for extra protein)

- 2 tablespoons of olive oil

- 1 cup shredded vegan cheese (optional)

Use a cooking pot of large size in heating up the olive oil before adding the chili pepper, garlic, black pepper, cumin, sea salt, and other spices. Cook on medium for 5 minutes, before adding the vegetables and sautéing for another six mins. Add in the tomatoes and paste, stirring and mixing the spices into the sauce. Drain and rinse all the beans and return it back inside the pot. Cook, stirring, for about fifteen mins in medium-heat setting, then reduce and cook for another hour, adding more spices as desired. Serve topped with cilantro or parsley, and/or vegan cheese (shredded).

Soy ground round or other vegan versions of ground "beef" can be added to thicken the chili, or in place of the textured vegetable protein, if used at all.

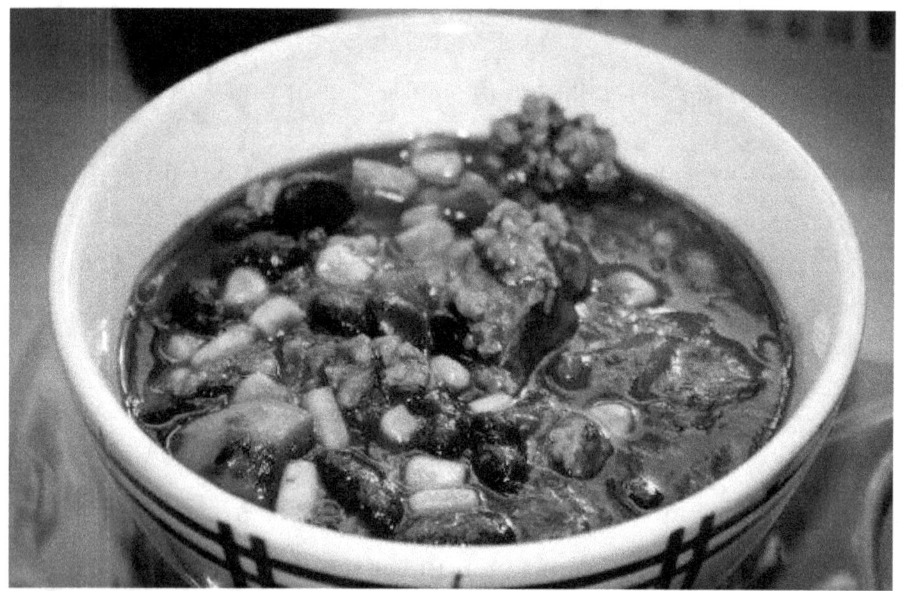

Spaghetti with Sauce and Baked Zucchini

A twist on a regular spaghetti and meat sauce dish, this meal uses baked zucchini as the central feature, served with the pasta sauce and noodles.

- 2 large zucchinis, sliced in half lengthwise
- 2 cans of crushed tomatoes
- ¼ cup of tomato paste
- 3 cloves of garlic, grated or crushed
- 1 teaspoon of black pepper
- 1 teaspoon of thyme
- 1 teaspoon of chili pepper
- 1 tablespoon of oregano
- Dash of sea salt
- ½ package of uncooked pasta noodles (spaghetti is recommended)
- ½ cup of vegan parmesan

Slice and rinse the zucchini, coat lightly in sea salt, and place on a baking dish lined with paper and in an oven that is already preheated to 350 degrees. Bake for 25-30 minutes. While the zucchini is in the oven, heat a medium or small skillet with olive oil and add in the oregano, chili pepper, black pepper, thyme, and sea salt. Cook for another 5-6 minutes, then add in the crushed garlic for a few more minutes until softened. Pour in the tomato paste and crushed tomatoes and reduce heat. Transfer to a large or medium cooking pot to continue stewing, if needed. In a separate cooking pot, boil up to four cups of water before adding in the pasta. Add 1 teaspoon of salt, reduce to medium, and cook until tender. Drain the spaghetti and set aside.

When the zucchini is baked, removed from the oven and place on a large oval serving dish. Scoop the spaghetti or pasta and add around the zucchini, then pour the pasta sauce over everything. Coat the top in vegan parmesan and serve. This dish serves 4-6 people and takes approximately one hour to prepare.

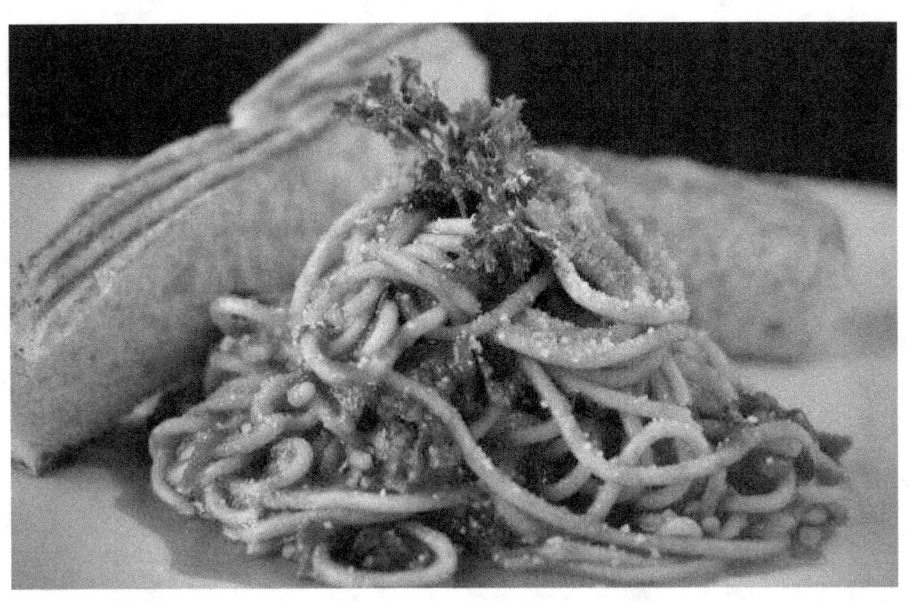

Veggie Burger Patties

If you crave burgers, these patties will provide the right fix. Served with or without a bun, these veggie burger patties can be a tasty meal on their own or as a traditional hamburger. The making of this recipe combines beans and mushrooms for a delicious mix.

- 1 small white or yellow onion, diced

- 3 green onions, sliced

- 1 teaspoon of cumin

- 1 cup of sliced mushrooms

- 1 tablespoon of olive oil

- 2 crushed cloves of garlic

- 1 cup of pinto beans

- 1 teaspoon of black pepper

- 1 teaspoon of dill or parsley

The olive oil should be heated first in a cooking pan before adding the garlic and the onions. Simmer on medium for 3-4 minutes. Add in the cumin, green onions, and mushrooms and continue to cook for another 5-6 minutes, or until the vegetables are tender. Reduce the heat to low to simmer, then remove from heat and set aside. Drain and rinse a can of pinto beans. Pour into a medium bowl and mash until they resemble refried beans. Beans can also be processed in a blender until smooth. Return the beans to the bowl and mix in the mushroom and onion mix from the skillet. Blend until smooth, then form into burger-sized patties and set aside. Heat a skillet on medium with olive oil. Lightly fry each side of each burger for about 3-4 minutes, or until browned, then serve.

Variations to this recipe include the following:

- Add one or two tablespoons of chili powder to make it spicy or one diced jalapeno pepper

- Replace pinto beans with black beans for a different taste, or combine both into the same portion

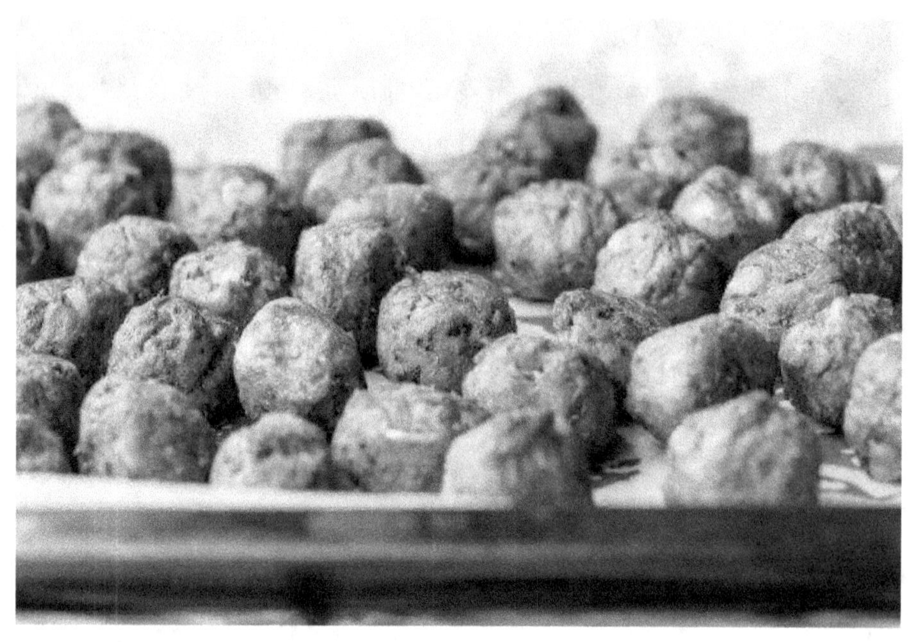

Tofu Scramble with Greens

This dish is often prepared for breakfast, though it can be prepared for any meal of the day. Firm tofu is marinated in a light broth and prepared the next morning. As with most marinades, the minimum recommended time to soak the tofu is two hours. The tofu can be prepared the night before and marinated overnight or two hours before your next meal. The ingredients are simple and easy to use:

- 1 teaspoon of black pepper

- 1 tablespoon of turmeric

- 1 teaspoon of sea salt

- 2 cups of vegetable broth

- ½ teaspoon of oregano

- ½ teaspoon of thyme

- ¼ teaspoon of tarragon

Combine the above ingredients in a small bowl to create the marinade. Drain and rinse one block of tofu and slice into cubes. Add to a small or medium container and pour the broth marinade to coat the tofu completely. If tofu is not completely covered, add more vegetable broth until it's submerged. Place in the refrigerator for two hours or longer, then rinse and retain ½ cup of the liquid in a small bowl.

To prepare the tofu, heat a skillet on medium with olive oil. Mash the tofu in a bowl until it is crumbly, then pour the ½ cup of leftover liquid and mix. Add to the skillet and fry. Sprinkle any spices you prefer, such as chili pepper, curry, and/or thyme. To add in the greens, choose spinach or arugula (one cup), then drain and rinse. Chop and add to the skillet. Continue to cook until tofu is gold or browned and greens are soft, then serve.

This is an excellent dish to get as many nutrients as possible with just a few ingredients. For a different twist on this dish, consider the following:

- Mix two tablespoons of coconut milk with one tablespoon of curry powder and mix it into the tofu scramble.

- Add two tablespoons of tomato paste and a few black beans. Serve with salsa and sliced avocado.

- Add a sliced jalapeno or green chili for a very spicy dish, then serve with vegan sour cream.

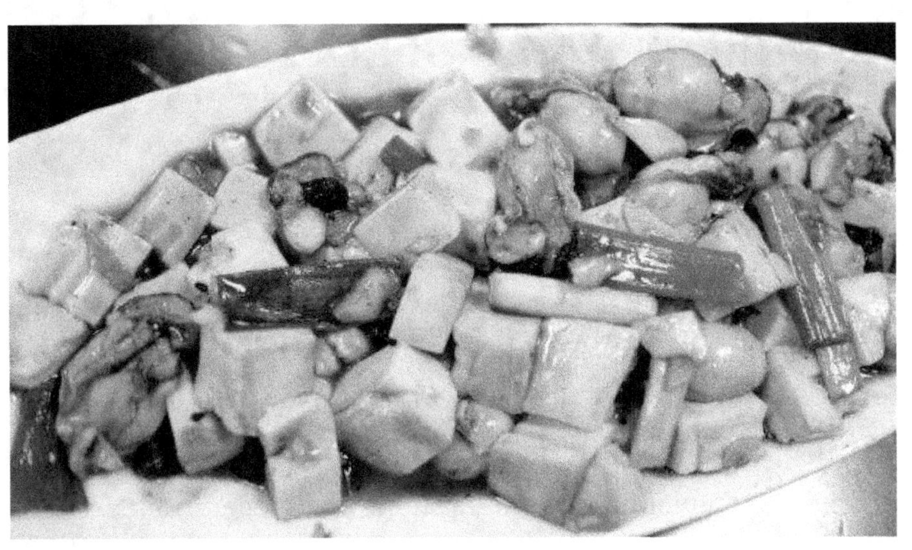

Chapter 6: 10 Snack Recipes

A vegan diet doesn't have to skip on snacks and tasty treats. There are plenty of plant-based ingredients that combine to make a wonderful assortment of bars, bite-sized treats. Consider some of the following recipes for planning your day. Packing one or two options will curb your temptation to choose sugary, high-fat snacks often offered in coffee shops and grocery stores.

Energy Bars

High protein and energy with low sugar and healthy fats, these bars are ideal to prepare for a workout or a busy day at the office. To make these bars, no baking or cooking is required. Chia seeds are an important ingredient, as they contain a wealth of nutrients, including fiber, protein, and antioxidants.

- 1 cup of pitted and sliced dates

- ½ cup of cocoa powder

- ½ cup of chia seeds

- 1 cup of crushed pistachios

- ½ cup of shredded coconut

- 1 teaspoon vanilla extract

- ½ cup of raw dark chocolate chips

- ¾ cups of raw oats

Use a food processor to smoothly blend the dates before adding the walnuts and continuing to blend. Pour the remaining items to pulse together until they are all evenly mixed. Remove and transfer the dough mixture to a small bowl and knead together, forming small, bar-shaped portions, and place on a lined baking tray. Place in the freezer for a minimum of two hours or overnight, then remove, slice, and serve.

These are delicious snacks and pack a lot of nutrients into each bite. To vary the recipe for a slightly different taste, consider the following options:

- Add 1 teaspoon of cinnamon or nutmeg

- Mix in 1 teaspoon of coconut oil

- Replace the pistachios with crushed walnuts, pecans, or slivered almonds

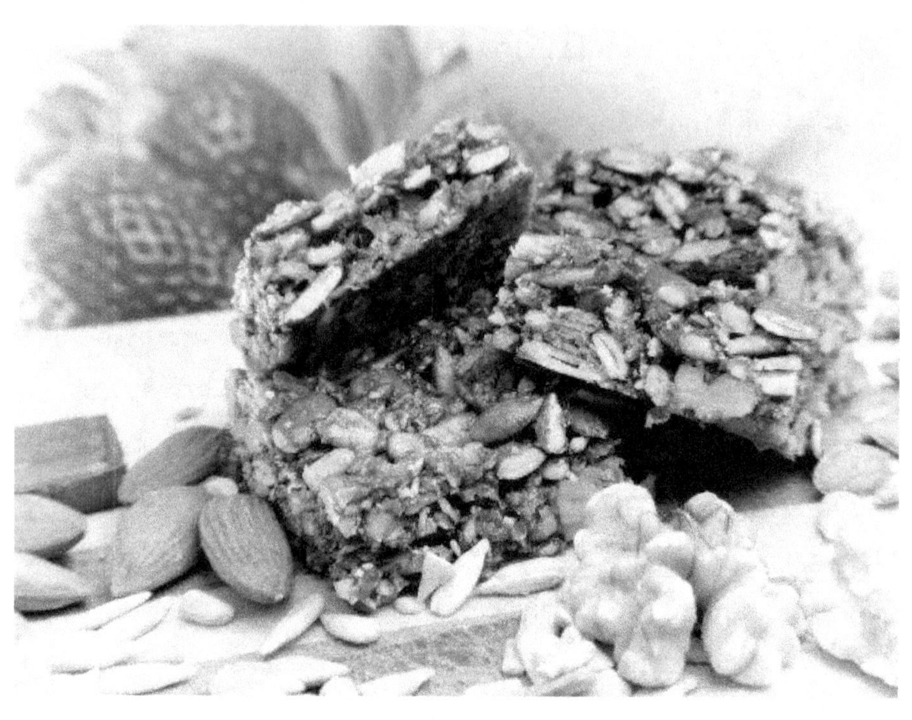

Peanut Butter and Chocolate Energy Bites

These are easy to make and minimal ingredient treats that are rolled into small, ball-sized servings. Usually, two or three can satisfy as a tasty snack in between meals. These are prepared using a small ice cube tray or silicone molds to form and freeze. No baking or cooking is required.

- 1 cup of peanut butter (sugar-free and unsalted)

- 2 tablespoons of raw oats

- 2 teaspoons of chia seeds

- 1 teaspoon of vanilla extract

- 2 tablespoons of cocoa powder

- 1 teaspoon of maple syrup

In a mixing dish of medium size, mix the peanut butter with the maple syrup until evenly mixed. Add in the cocoa powder and vanilla extra, mashing until the cocoa is completely coating the peanut butter mix, then add in the raw oats and chia seeds, using your hands to completely combine the ingredients. Form the dough into balls and add to silicone molds or an ice cube tray and freeze for one hour, then move the refrigerator. These treats can be kept up to one week in the refrigerator or a month in the freezer. This recipe makes about 4-5 servings and takes only 5-6 minutes to prepare.

For a slight variation, replace the peanut butter with tahini or almond butter. If replacing with tahini, adding a teaspoon of raw or toasted sesame seeds is another option.

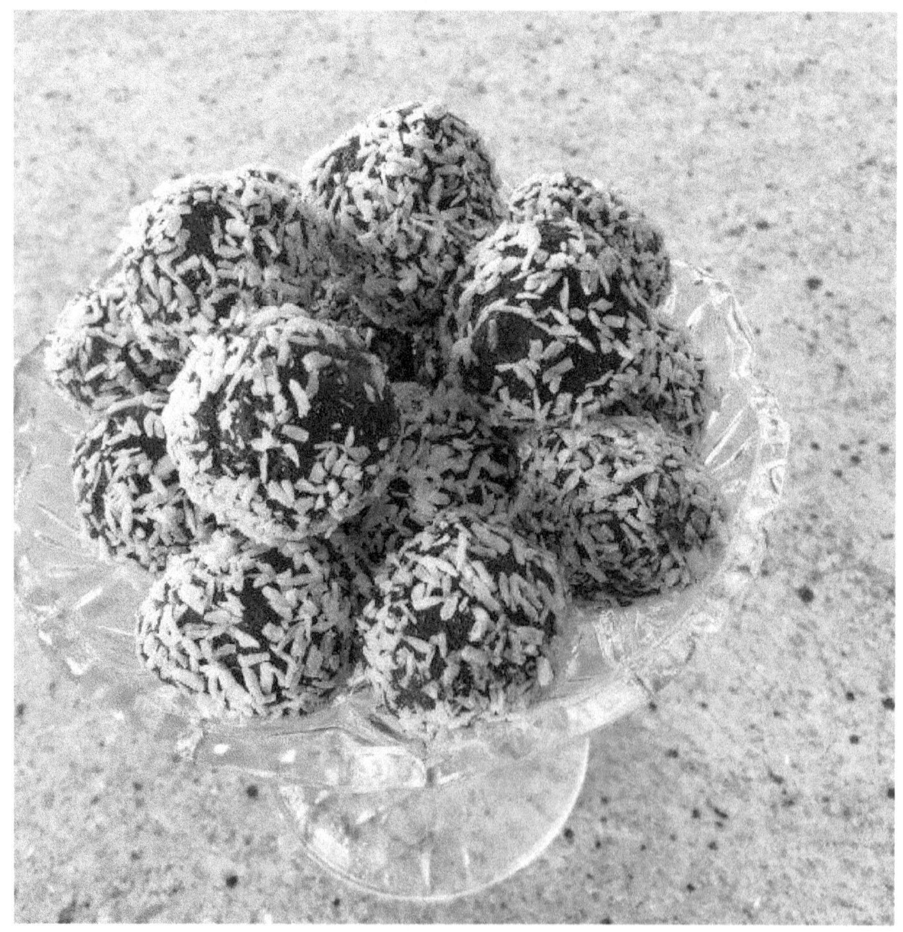

Pistachio and Cardamom Treats

This treat is created like fat bombs, which are healthy fat treats infused with a large selection or combination of flavors. In this recipe, cardamom and pistachios are combined with coconut oil to create small, bite-sized fat bombs, which are stored in the freezer for two hours before serving.

- 3 tablespoons of coconut oil, melted at room temperature

- ½ teaspoons crushed cardamom pods or powder

- 1 teaspoon of maple syrup

- 2-3 tablespoons of crushed pistachios

Blend the entire ingredients together into a small bowl and pour into silicone molds or an ice cube tray. Freeze for at least two hours before servings. Keep frozen until ready to serve. This recipe makes enough for 4-5.

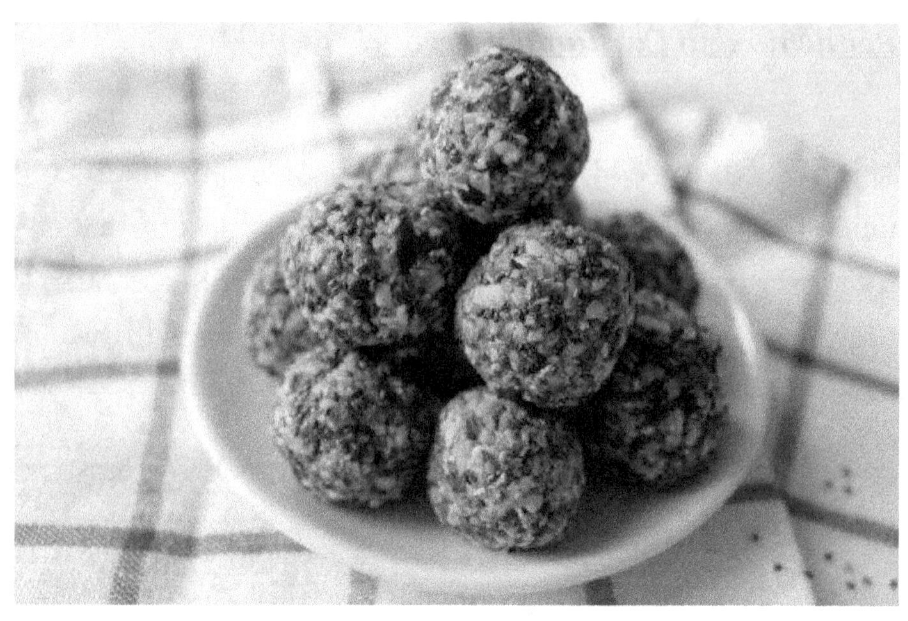

Lemon-Lime Cheesecake Cupcake Fat Bombs

Inspired by key lime pie and cheesecake, this vegan version and fat bomb version is tasty and much easier to make.

- 1 teaspoon of low carb sweetener

- 2 teaspoons of lemon juice

- 2 teaspoons of lime juice

- ½ cup of vegan cream cheese

Mix all ingredients in a small mixing dish and pour into silicone molds or an ice cube tray. Freeze for two hours and serve. Makes enough for 4-5 servings.

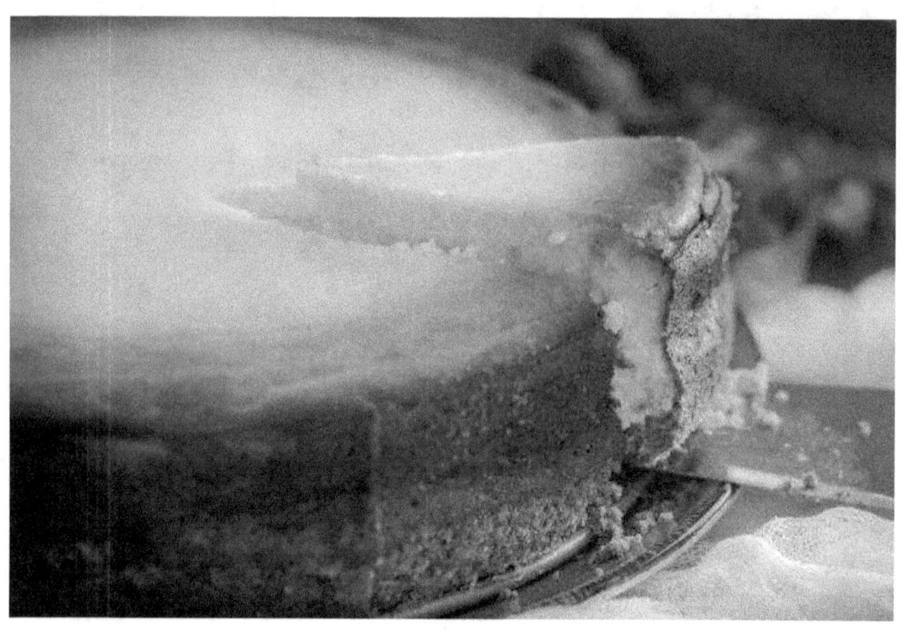

Macaroons

These treats are an ideal blend of coconut and cocoa or dark chocolate. Only a few ingredients are needed to make these no-bake macaroons.

- 1/3 cup of coconut oil

- 1 cup of shredded coconut

- 5 tablespoons of cocoa powder

- 1 teaspoon of vanilla or almond extract

- 3 cups of raw oats

- 2 tablespoons maple syrup

- ½ cups of coconut milk

Combine the coconut milk, oil, vanilla or almond extract, and maple syrup into a bowl and stir together. In a different container, combine the cocoa powder, shredded coconut, and raw oats. Combine both bowls of ingredients and form into balls. Refrigerate for at least two hours before servings.

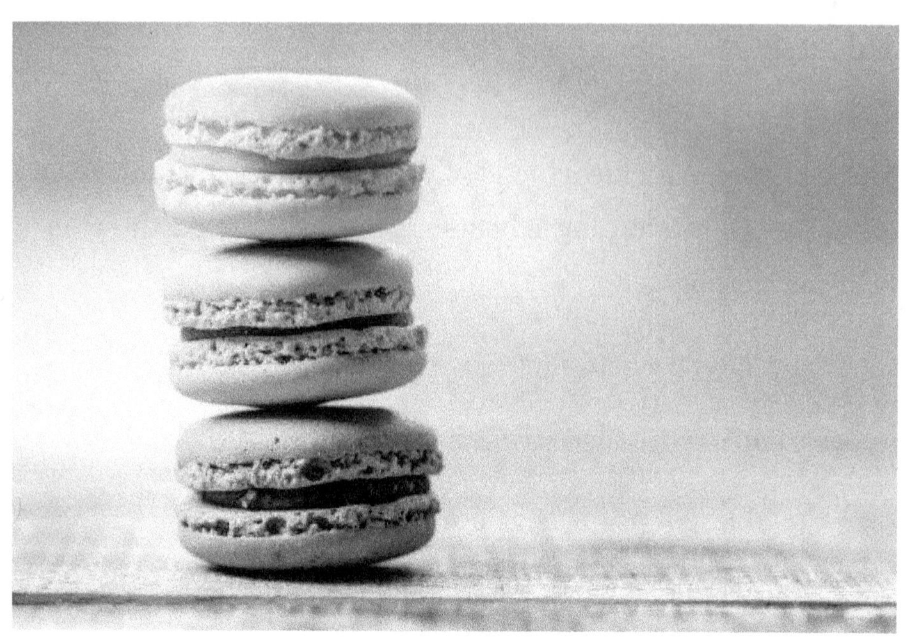

Easy Plant-Based Snacks

Kale Chips

Kale chips are often expensive in specialty grocery and natural food stores, though they are budget-friendly and healthier to make at home. They can be prepared in less than 15 minutes and baked in only 10 minutes, which makes them a quick and easy snack to make. Only three ingredients are needed:

- 2 tablespoons of olive oil

- 1 tablespoon of sea salt

- 1 bunch of kale

Wash and drain one bunch of kale, then remove stems and slice into one or two-inch pieces (chip or bite-sized). Lightly coat each kale piece in olive oil, and place on a large, lined baking sheet. Sprinkle each kale slice with sea salt and preheat the oven, setting to 350 degrees. Bake for 8-10 minutes or until crispy, but not burnt.

Spicy Kale Chips

This recipe involves using one of two spices to create a strong but tasty version of baked kale chips:

- 2 tablespoons of olive oil

- Dash of salt

- 1 teaspoon of cayenne pepper

- 1 teaspoon of chili powder

- 1 bunch of kale

Mix the salt, chili powder, and cayenne powder together, and set aside. Prepare the kale as the recipe above. Use olive oil in coating the kale lightly. Sprinkle a mixture of pepper and salt. Bake for 8-10 minutes and serve. There is the option to skip salt completely and simply use cayenne and/or the chili pepper options.

"Cheesy" Kale Chips

If you enjoy vegan parmesan "cheese", this version of kale chips can be a fun option to try making.

- ½ teaspoons of sea salt

- 2 tablespoons of olive oil

- 1 bunch of kale

- 2 tablespoons of vegan parmesan "cheese"

Prepare the kale like the previous recipes and coat with the olive oil. Place the kale slices on the lined baking tray, and sprinkle salt, then coat with parmesan. Bake for slightly longer, 10-11 minutes, until slightly brown or gold, then remove from the oven and serve.

Roasted Chickpeas

Chickpeas are a great snack to enjoy raw, cooked, or baked into a crispy chip. This recipe provides an easy way to create roasted chickpeas with minimal ingredients.

- ½ of a can of chickpeas

- ½ teaspoon of chili powder (optional)

- 1 teaspoon of salt

- 2 tablespoons of olive oil

Drain and rinse the chickpeas and dry, then pour into a bowl. Lightly coat all chickpeas in olive oil, then mix the chili powder and sea salt together, and coat the beans. Transfer the chickpeas to a lined baking tray and bake for 20-25 minutes on 350 degrees.

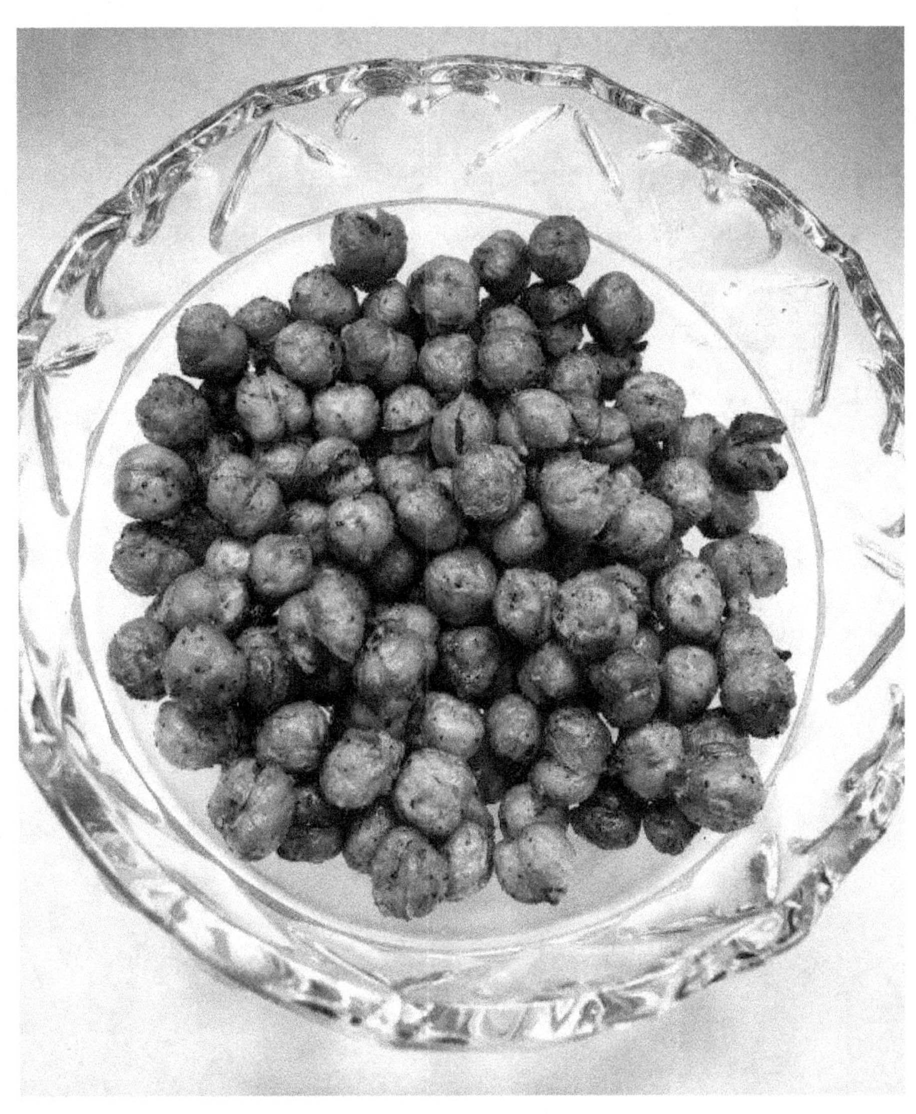

Cinnamon Roasted Pumpkin Seeds

Don't throw away the pumpkin seeds after using a pumpkin for carving or another recipe. The seeds offer a great snack opportunity. Most roasted pumpkin seeds are prepared with salt, though this treat combines cinnamon, instead, for a sweet and savory treat.

- 1 cup of raw pumpkin seeds

- 2 teaspoons of cinnamon

- 2 teaspoons of coconut oil or olive oil

Coat all the pumpkin seeds in olive or coconut oil and arrange on a large baking tray. Sprinkle evenly with cinnamon and bake for 20-25 minutes until slightly crispy, but not burnt.

Chapter 7: 10 Dessert Recipes

Puddings and Yogurt-based Desserts

Vegan or non-dairy yogurt and puddings are delicious options for dessert in plant-based eating. The following recipes are light and tasty, without the guilt of high fats and sugars or dairy products.

Rice Pudding

This recipe uses coconut milk as a creamy foundation for a rich dessert and avoids dairy completely. Basmati rice is used for its nutty, aromatic flavor, and how it blends well with the other ingredients in this recipe.

- 1 cup of basmati rice (uncooked)

- 4 cans of coconut milk (unsweetened) or 6 measured cups

- 1 ½ cups of low carb sweetener (monk fruit or swerve is recommended)

- 1 teaspoon of vanilla extract

- 1 cup of water

- 2 tablespoons of coconut oil or butter

- Cinnamon for the topping

In a large cooking pot, combine the coconut milk, basmati rice, sweetener, and water, and bring to a boil, then reduce heat and continue to cook and simmer for about one hour. Add in the vanilla extract and simmer, stirring regularly until the mixture thickens. Add in the coconut butter or oil and simmer a few more minutes, then remove from heat to cool. Serve sprinkled with cinnamon.

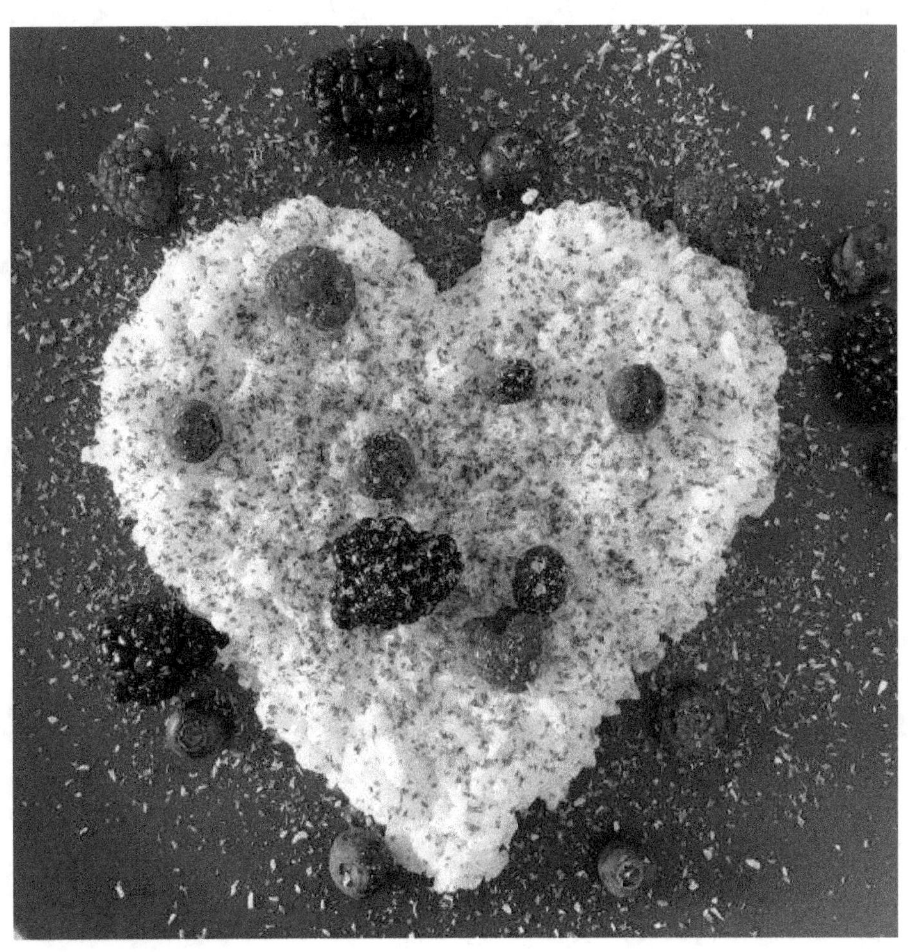

Chia Seed Pudding

If you want a dessert that's healthy and as a meal at the same time, chia seed pudding is the solution. This recipe involves mixing chia seeds with coconut milk, cream, and a variety of toppings for a fun treat, which also provides essential vitamins, protein, and fiber. When chia seeds are soaked in milk or liquid, they become soft and custard-like, which makes them ideal for creating puddings and parfaits.

- 1 cup of chia seeds

- 2 cup of coconut milk

- 2 teaspoons coconut cream or butter

- 1 teaspoon of vanilla extract

- ¼ cup of sweetener (low carb sweetener or maple syrup)

In a small container or bowl, whisk together all the above ingredients. Chia seeds tend to stick to utensils, and it may take a few minutes to thoroughly blends everything. Store in the refrigerator for two hours or more, then remove to serve. The pudding should have a thick, custard-like consistency that is easy to scoop and serve. This recipe serves 2-3 and takes only a few minutes to prepare, before chilling in the refrigerator.

Note: Refrigerating the chia seed pudding overnight allows for the option of enjoying this dessert as breakfast the next morning.

Topping options for this treatment include:

- Cocoa powder or chocolate chips (dark chocolate is recommended)

- Cardamom powder

- Crushed nuts, such as peanuts, pistachios, slivered almonds, crushed pecans, etc.

- Fresh fruits sliced: berries, bananas, melon, peaches, mangos, pineapples, etc.

- Shredded coconut

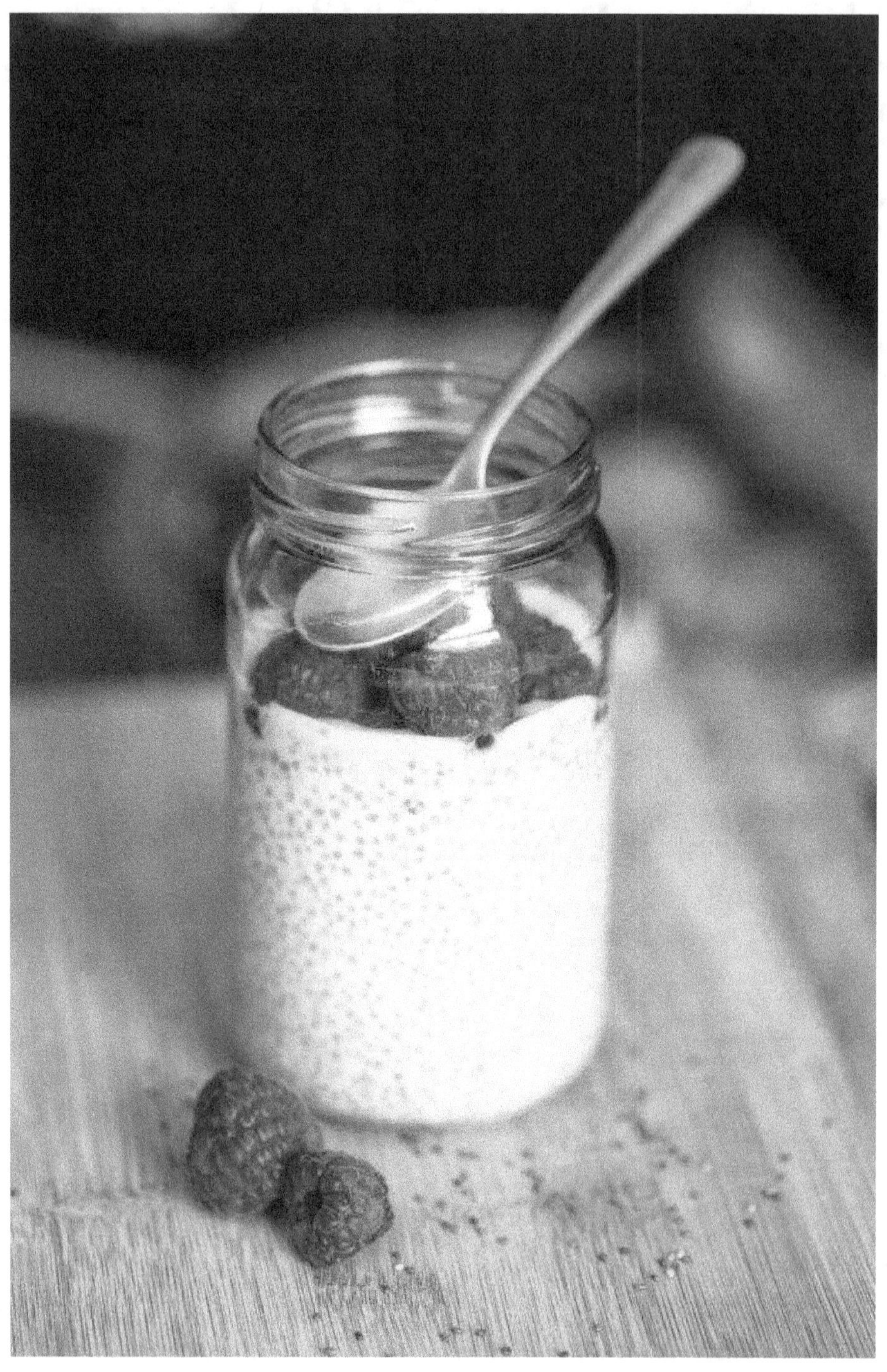

Coconut Yogurt Parfait

The vegan yogurt included in this recipe is made of cultured coconut and can be used in the exact same way as regular, dairy yogurt for this treat.

- ½ cup of crushed peanuts

- 1 cup of sliced berries

- 2 cups of coconut yogurt

- 2 tablespoons of maple syrup

- 2 tablespoons of chocolate chips

- ½ cup of raw oats

In a large sundae glass, add the sliced fruits at the bottom, then scoop heaving spoonful amounts of the coconut yogurt on top and mixing in some of the chocolate chips and maple syrup. On the top layer, top with crushed peanuts oats.

Chia seeds, hemp seeds, and flax can be added to this dish to add more nutrients and protein.

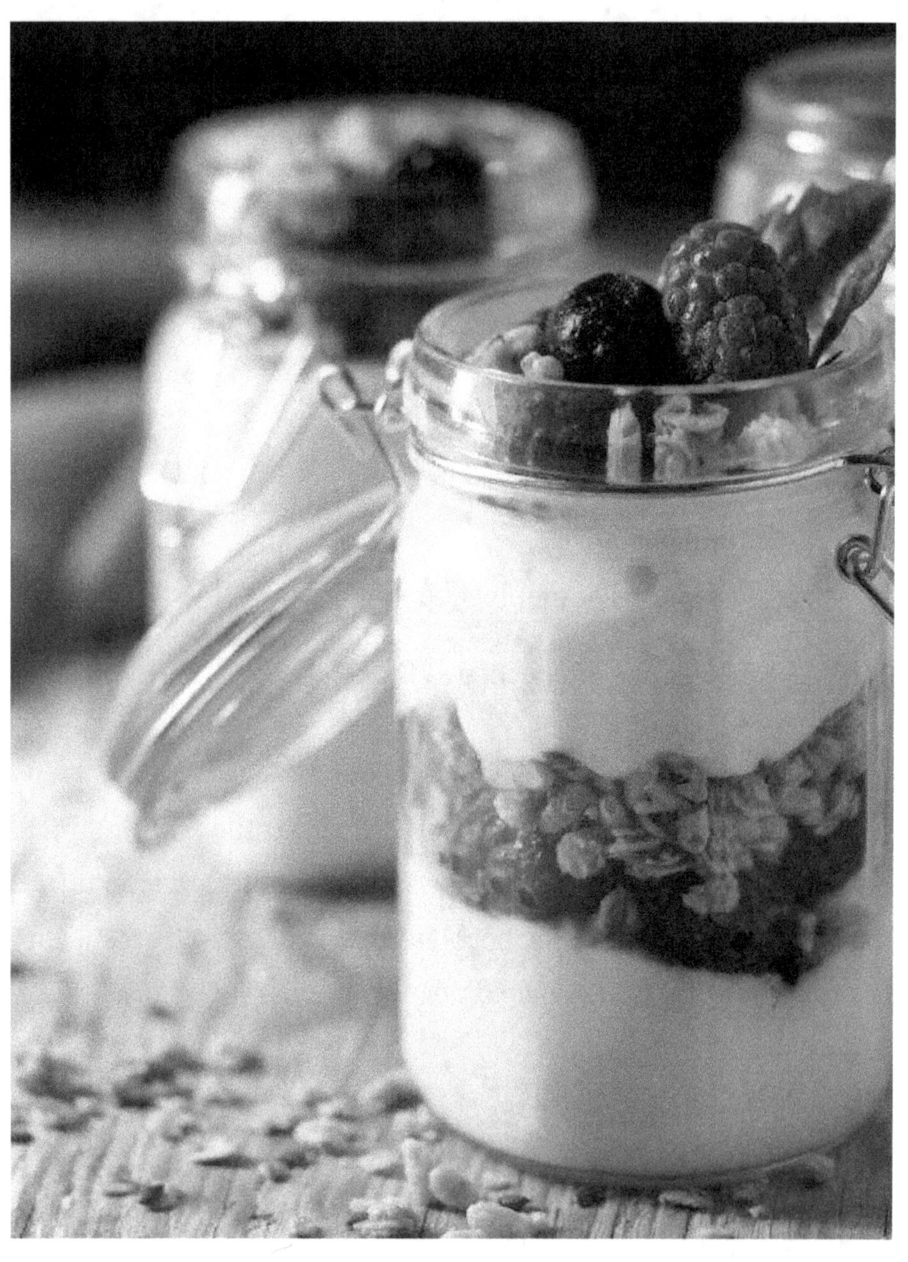

**Sticky Rice and Mango Dessert**

This dish involves cooking sticky rice with coconut and layering a baking pan, then topped with fresh mango. This dessert is light and refreshing and a good way to finish a meal.

- 2 sliced mangoes (pits removed, sliced)

- 2 cups of sticky rice (uncooked)

- 2 tablespoons of low carb sweetener or maple syrup

- 1 cup of water

- 3 cups of coconut milk

- 1 teaspoon of sesame seeds

Add the water and coconut milk to a cooking pot and bring to a bowl on medium heat. Add in the rice and cook until tender and "sticky". Remove from heat and pour into a large or medium-sized baking dish, making sure the rice evenly coats the bottom of the pan. Cool for 20-25 minutes, then layer the sliced mangoes over the rice, ensuring they cover the entire surface (add more mango if needed). Sprinkle the sesame seeds over the mangoes and serve. If mangoes are not available, peaches make a great substitute.

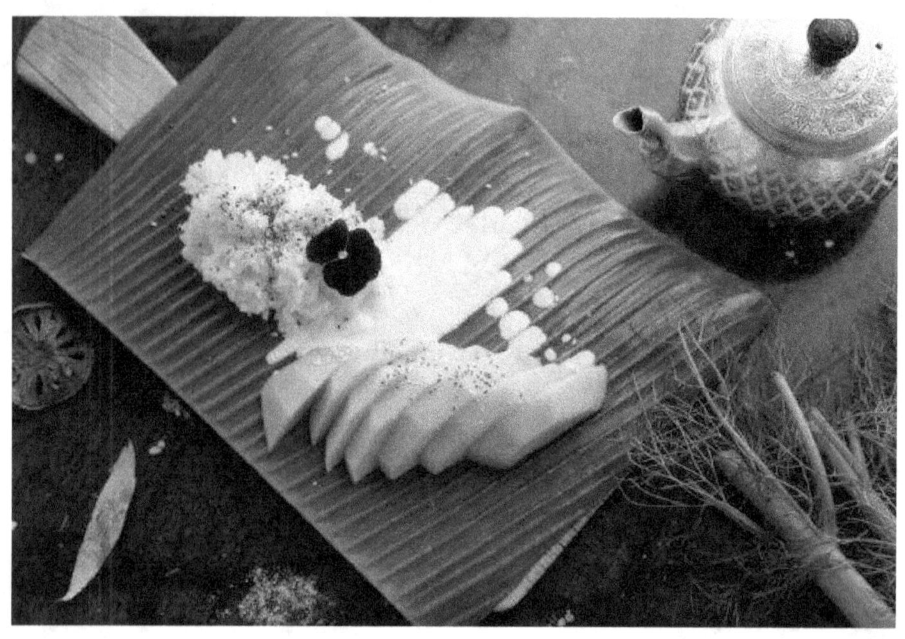

Sweet Potato and Pumpkin Pudding

A sweet and tasty treat, sweet potato pudding can also satisfy an appetite like a main dish and is full of nutrients, such as beta carotene and fiber.

- 1/3 cups of rolled oats

- 1 large cooked sweet potato or yam (baked)

- 1 tablespoon of maple syrup

- 1 teaspoon of cinnamon

- 2 tablespoons of pumpkin puree

- ½ cup of soy or almond milk

Mix the entire ingredients listed above in a blender until it has a smooth consistency. Serves 2-3 and takes only 10 minutes to prepare (not including baking the yam, which can take up to one hour).

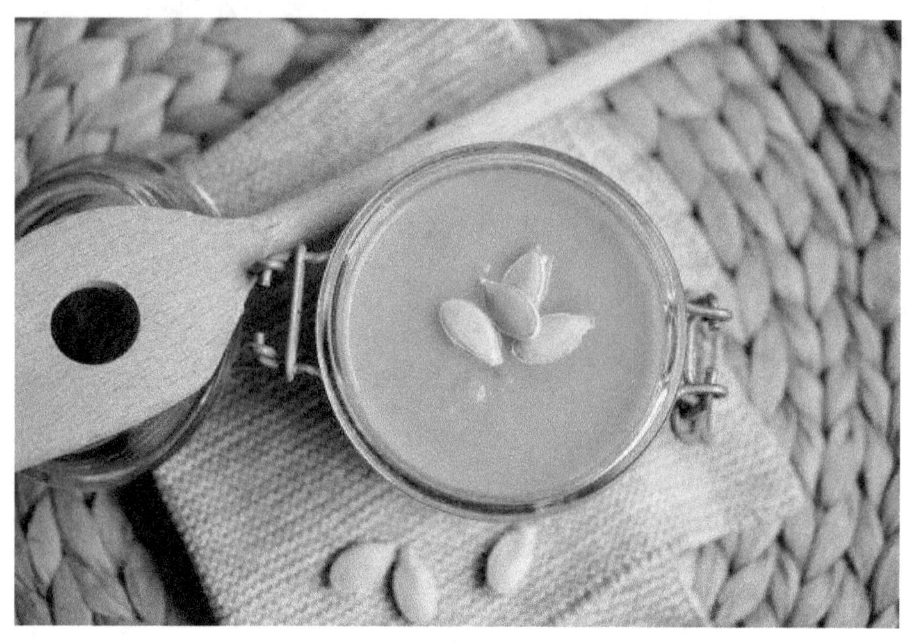

Sweet and Sour Rhubarb Yoghurt Parfait

This recipe is like the regular coconut yogurt parfait, with the addition of stewed rhubarb, which provides a sweet and sour flavor combination.

- 1 cup of blueberries

- 1 cup of stewed rhubarb

- 2 cups of coconut yogurt

- 2 teaspoons of maple syrup

- ½ cups of chia seeds

- ¼ cups of rolled oats

To prepare the rhubarb, slice 2-3 stalks into one-inch pieces before adding in a casserole full of water. Let it start boiling before adding in 2 teaspoons of maple syrup, then reduce in heat and continue to cook on medium until the rhubarb is soft. Remove, drain, and rinse, then place in a bowl to be chilled for almost half an hour.

In a large dessert cup or sundae glass, scoop the rhubarb to the bottom of the cup, then top with several scoops of coconut yogurt, swirling in the maple syrup, then top with the chia seeds, blueberries, and rolled oats. For best results, soak the chia seeds in coconut milk or yogurt of two hours before adding to this recipe.

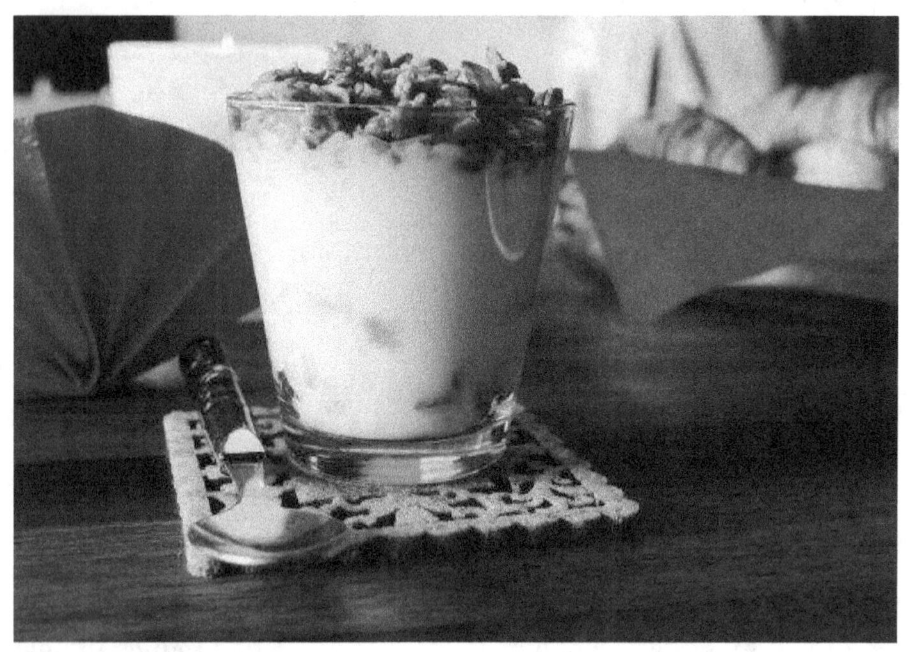

Cakes

Brownie Cake

This vegan chocolate cake resembles a large decadent brownie with a rich texture. It's the ultimate comfort food and made with all plant-based ingredients.

- 1 cup of low carb sweetener (monk fruit or swerve)

- 1 tablespoon coconut flour

- 2 cups of almond flour

- Dash of sea salt

- 1 cup of cocoa powder of baker's chocolate

- ½ cup of coconut oil

- 1 cup of water

- 1 teaspoon of baking powder

- 1 teaspoon of vanilla extract

Mix all the dry ingredients in a large bowl and set aside. Prepare the oven by setting it to 350 degrees. Pour the following items into the bowl with the cocoa, flours, and sweetener: water, coconut oil, and vanilla extract. Blend thoroughly, then pour into a lined or greased baking pan, and bake for 25-30 minutes.

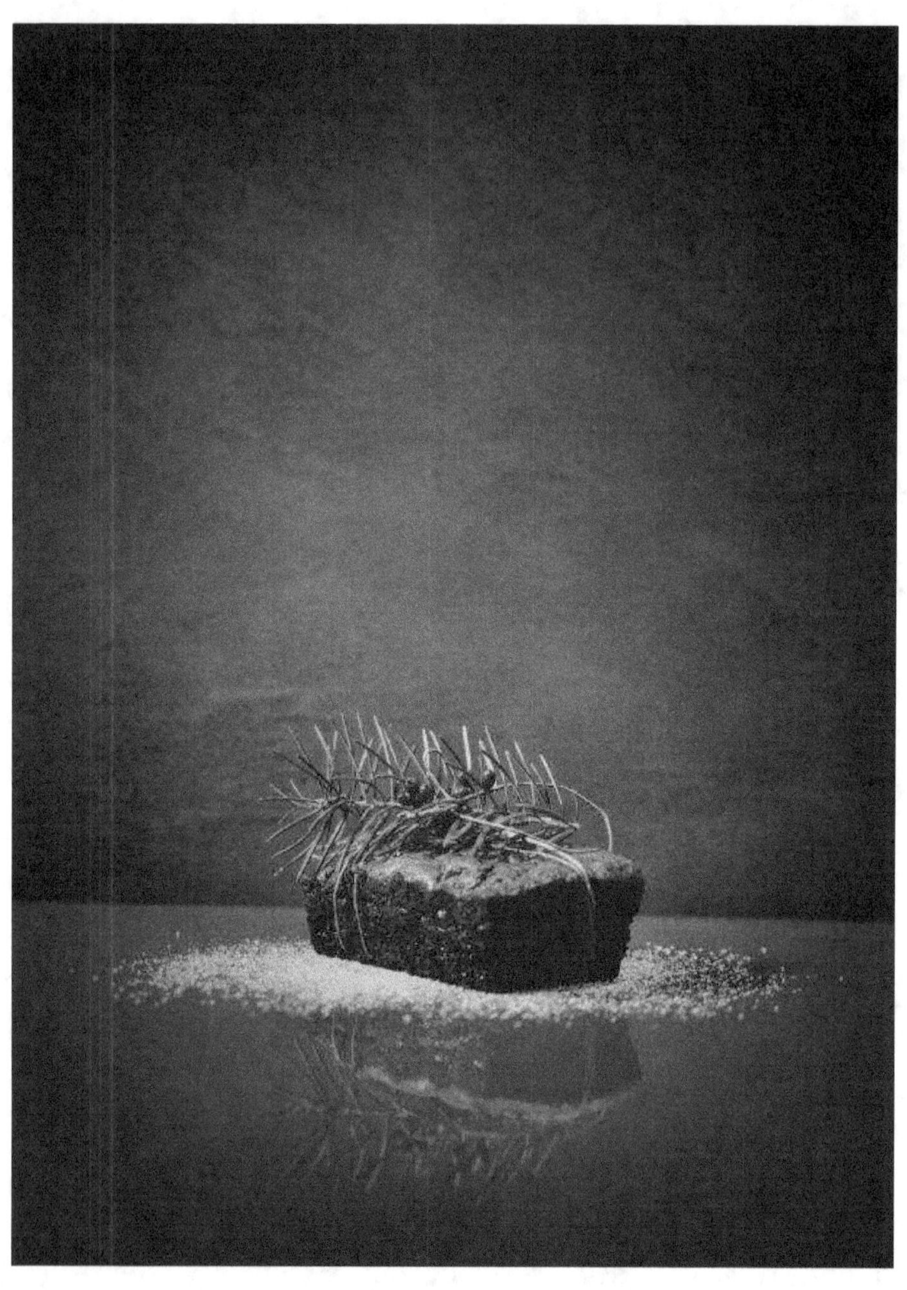

Vanilla Cake

This is a basic cake recipe that can provide a platform for many toppings, syrups, and fruit options. To prepare this cake, combine the dry and wet ingredients in separate bowls, then mix together to bake:

- 1 teaspoon of vanilla extract

- 1 tablespoon apple cider vinegar

- 1 ½ cups of coconut or almond milk

- ½ cup of applesauce (unsweetened)

Combine the above ingredients into a medium bowl, then set aside. Prepare the oven by preheating to 350 degrees. Mix the following ingredient separately in a medium bowl:

- 3 cups of almond flour

- 1 cup of potato starch

- 1 cup of low carb sweetener (monk fruit or swerve)

- 1 teaspoon of baking powder

- 1 teaspoon of baking soda

- Dash of sea salt

- ½ cup of cornstarch

Mix both sets of ingredients together in the larger bowl and prepare a lined cake tin for the oven. Place on a dish ideal for baking before cooking in the oven for about a quarter of an hour or until lightly brown or golden on top. Chill for 10-15 minutes, then serve.

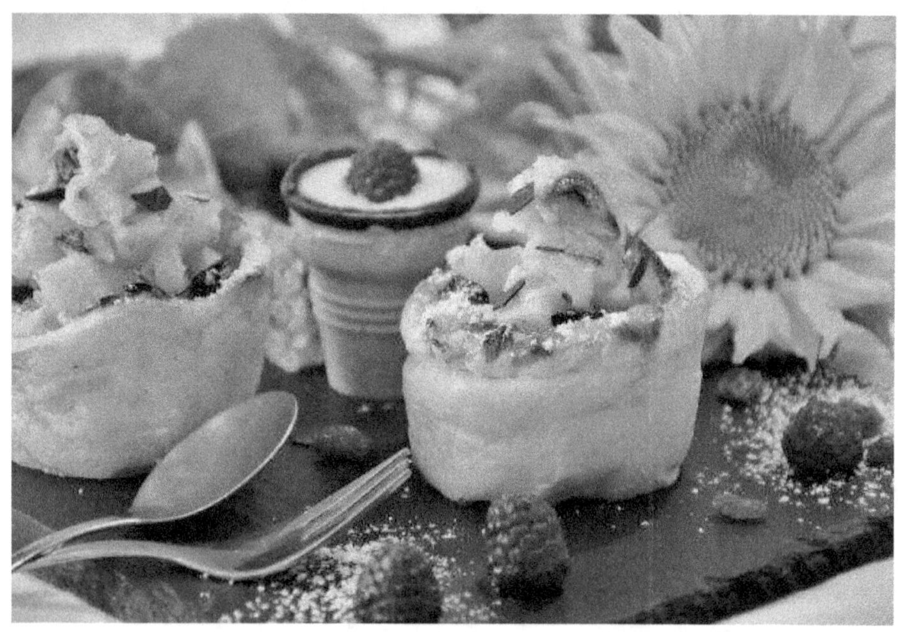

Chapter 8: Starting Your Weight Loss Program: A Four-Week Plan

Weekly Plans and Meals for Each Day of the Week, for Four Weeks

If you're new to a plant-based diet, this four-week plan will give you the tools to start on the right track. During the next four weeks, following these meal plans can help you incorporate a new series of recipes, as well as easy plant-based eating, into an easy-to-follow plan that can set a good foundation for future choices. Getting acquainted with healthy, plant-based foods means incorporating them into your everyday life, so they can be of benefit to you on a regular basis. These plans are also excellent for planning your shopping trips and making choices about the fruits, vegetables, nuts, seeds, soy products, and other foods you select.

Week 1: Plant-based Diet Plan

During your first week, try lots of new and different recipes, or try just a few. Smoothies for breakfast offer a fast and nutritious way to get what you need quickly so that you can move into your day without having to clean up much. Many of the lunch and dinner options are easy to prepare and can be made the night before to make the planning easier. Consider the possibility of leftovers from the lunch or dinner yesterday, and use them the following day, or freeze and/or refrigerate for later in the week. Snacks and desserts are added as an option, though they can be changed or skipped completely if desired.

Week 1	Mon	Tues	Wed	Thurs	Fri	Sat	Sun
Breakfast	Kiwi-Banana and Strawberry Smoothie	Chia seed pudding	Avocado Banana Smoothie	Pumpkin Cinnamon Smoothie	Coconut Yogurt Berry Smoothie	Scrambled Tofu with spinach	Chia seed pudding with fresh fruit
Lunch	Kale and Blueberry salad	Butternut squash soup with rye bread	Lentil dal	Leftover tempeh with yogurt	Green pea soup	Spinach, mandarin and walnut salad	Curried chickpeas
Snack	Apple	Sliced avocado	Hummus on toast	Chocolate brownie	Chia seed pudding	Sliced mangos with peanuts	Black olives with celery sticks

Dinner	Baked tofu	Veggie skillet dish	Sweet and sour tempeh	Tofu, roasted squash, and miso soup	Veggie burgers	Quinoa salad	Veggie skillet dish
Dessert	Yogurt parfait with rhubarb and berries	Fruit salad	Slice of brownie cake	An apple	Sweet and sour tempeh	Zucchini with pasta sauce and noodles	Vanilla cake

Week 2: Plant-based Diet Plan

During your second week, you may notice a difference in the way you feel and eat. You may experience more energy and want to explore new foods or continue to use a lot of the recipes during the first week. Choosing new ingredients or switching them (for example, adding different fruits or combinations of fruits to smoothies) is one way to try something new. Enjoying a baked tofu dinner with vegetables may result in leftover tofu that can be added to a salad or soup the next day. Not only will this help add a variety of different flavors to each meal, but it will also save money on how the foods are used and incorporated into your diet.

Week 1	Mon	Tues	Wed	Thurs	Fri	Sat	Sun
Breakfast	Tropical smoothie	Fruit salad and peanut butter energy bites	Scrambled tofu with arugula	Fruit salad with yogurt	Pumpkin and cinnamon smoothie	Coconut yogurt with sliced banana	Chia seed pudding
Lunch	Miso soup with avocado toast	Cup of chili	Arugula and roasted pear salad	Roasted eggplant with hummus on rye	Toasted rye with avocado	Lentil dal	Leftover lentil dal with a dollop of yogurt
Snack	An orange	A handful of roasted almonds	Rice pudding	Banana	A glass of soymilk with cocoa powder	Kale chips	Fresh fruit bowl
Dinner	Green pea soup		Tofu bake with squash	Stir-fried tempeh with vegetables and rice		Curried chickpeas and sautéed	Sweet ad sour tempeh

						onion s	
Desse rt	Brow nie cake	Vanil la cake	Mang o and cocon ut sticky rice desser t	Bana na and a slice of vanill a cake	Leftov er brown ie slice	Fruit salad	Rice pudd ing

Week 3: Plant-based Diet Plan

By the third week, you'll become more familiar with how to prepare for grocery shopping and which foods to select. Most people tend to favor certain foods and their flavors over others, and while this is normal, it's also a good idea to continue trying new vegetables, fruits, nuts, and seeds to get a better sense of what's available. All too often, people focus on the limitations of a diet rather than the opportunities available, especially when it comes to a plant-based diet. Eliminating meat and animal byproducts doesn't have to be expensive or restrictive if you're open to trying a wide range of foods and meal options.

Week 1	Mon	Tue s	Wed	Thurs	Fri	Sat	Sun
Break fast	Pumpk in Cinna mon	Yog urt wit h fres	Chia seed puddi ng	Mang o and pistac hio	Tofu scram ble with	Chia seed puddi ng with	Sliced apple s, spina ch,

	smoothie	h fruits		smoothie	sliced apple	chocolate chips	and crush walnuts and peanuts
Lunch	Ginger carrot soup	Veggie skillet meal	Kale blueberry salad	Stir-fried snow peas and slivered almonds	Baked tofu	Spinach salad with roasted pear	Baked tofu with sweet and sour sauce and rice
Snack	Sliced avocado	Kale chips	Spicy kale chips	Roasted chickpeas	Banana	Sliced apples and/or pears	Roasted chickpeas
Dinner	Miso soup with button mushrooms	Baked tofu with bok choy	Curried coconut with tofu and vegetables		Zucchini pasta dinner	Leftover pasta	Vegan chili
Dessert	Fresh fruit	Vanilla cake		Rice pudding	Rice pudding with pineapple	Brownie cake	

				and shredded coconut	

Week 4: Plant-based Diet Plan

In the final week, you will likely notice weight loss, even if you didn't expect to! A plant-based diet is low in calories, trans fats, and high in healthy fats, fiber, and protein, all of which keep your weight well-maintained and within a healthy level. At this stage, you may already be set up or planning your next week, using foods from this four-week plan and more. Always opt for new and exciting foods. Check out specialty shops where exotic fruits and vegetables are an option. Make a point of trying at least one new food each week or every two weeks, and you may find your preferences for food, and your palate will expand over time.

Week 1	Mon	Tues	Wed	Thurs	Fri	Sat	Sun
Breakfast	Banana and berry smoothie	Mango and pistachio smoothie	Chia seed pudding	Cherries and peaches smoothie	Chia seed pudding with sliced pineapple and shredded coconut	Avocado banana smoothie	Tofu scramble

Lunch	Lentil dal with burgers	Green pea soup	Lentil dal	Curried carrot and ginger soup	Veggie burger on a bun	Curried cabbage	Sweet and sour tempeh
Snack	Roasted pumpkin seeds	Roasted chickpeas	Banana	Spicy kale chips	A handful of ripe berries	Sliced avocado	Roasted chickpeas
Dinner	Tofu bake and squash	Tofu bake with quinoa salad	Vegetable wrap with tofu, and fresh vegetables	Avocado toast	Curried chickpeas	Lentil dal	Green pea soup
Dessert	Vanilla cake		Brownie cake		Yogurt with berries	Rice pudding	Chia seed pudding with cinnamon

Chapter 9: Conclusion

The plant-based diet offers a wide variety of options for meal preparation. Whether you're a beginner or more experienced with vegan eating, there are major benefits for weight loss and health overall. Choosing plant-based is an ethical and rewarding way of eating that will help you lose excess weight and maintain it at a healthy level. It's more than a diet, but rather, a long-term goal of eating and living well that can significantly improve your life.

Frequently Asked Questions

Question: Is it more expensive to follow a plant-based diet?

Answer: It depends on the food you choose that determines how expensive a vegan diet is. For example, if you eat a lot of prepared foods, such as pre-made salads and specialty foods, such as flavored tofu and/or other items that are outside of the regular whole foods, the price can increase significantly. Unfortunately, fresh produce can be expensive in some regions where it must be shipped and there are limited options, though in general, eating vegan should not cost a fortune. Reviewing the basic foods included in a plant-based diet and selecting the least expensive can help:

- Beans, legumes, and grains can be purchased in bulk or inconvenient cans at a decent price.

- Fresh vegetables and fruits can be expensive, though choosing a frozen option may be more convenient and less costly.

- Since meat and dairy are avoided, and these foods can add up to cost a lot, the only additional expense on your grocery bill are soy-based and other vegan foods that replace meat and dairy. The cost can range, though often, there are less expensive options available that make it easy for everyone.

- Nuts and seeds can be pricy for anyone, though buying in bulk is one way to focus on only the amounts you need while keeping within a budget.

Question: Is the vegan diet good for athletes?

Answer: Absolutely! In fact, you'll likely get more protein, calcium, and nutrients in general on a vegan diet. Choosing dark leafy green vegetables provides a wealth of vitamins, fiber, and protein that a lot of meat doesn't contain, and your body will metabolize and process plant-based foods easier, making weight loss success and getting into good shape a goal that can be achieved with the right commitment. There are a growing number of famous athletes and celebrities who adhere to a vegan diet with excellent results.

Question: How do I know if some of the foods I buy or choose are animal-free?

Answer: Choosing fresh fruits and vegetables is a surefire way to avoiding any meat products, as well as any other foods that are purchased in their whole form, including nuts, seeds, herbs, and spices. Tofu is soybean-based and almost never contains any meat or animal byproducts. To be certain, read all labels on the food items you buy, as many will have a label or sticker that notes if they are vegan, gluten-free, and/or nut-free. These labels are especially helpful for people who have allergies and need to avoid certain types of foods and ingredients.

Question: Are there any dangers of going vegan, such as vitamin or nutrient deficiencies or other conditions?

Answer: Fortunately, all your required nutrients can be easily consumed and included in a plant-based diet. This includes B12 and vitamin D. Vitamin B12 is found in fermented soy, such as miso and tempeh, as well as brewer's yeast. Vitamin D is absorbed through our skin from the sun, though it is also available in fortified milk and non-dairy milk beverages. Adequate amounts of protein, calcium, iron, and all other nutrient requirements are found in a wide range of plant-based foods. At one time, many people avoided eating vegan out of fear they would lose nutrients, which is quite the opposite. In fact, you'll find you're getting more out of a vegan or plant-based diet than if you choose meat and dairy.

Question: Should I switch my body care products, such as soaps, shampoos, moisturizers, and other items to vegan and cruelty-free options?

Answer: As a part of the vegan lifestyle, this is an excellent option, and there are a growing number of retailers who promote and design cruelty-free makeup, lotions, skincare, and body care products. This can extend to many other products, including lines of clothing and materials used in making a variety of items, including furniture. While some of these product lines can be expensive, some people who want a completely animal-free life can opt to choose these options as well. You may find that some vegan products, especially for body and skin, may be easier on your body and with less irritation or negative effects. As with any type of product, it's best to try them first, to determine if its right for you and your life, before continuing to use it.

Question: If I'm gluten intolerant or have Celiac disease, can I follow a vegan diet?

Answer: Yes, and it might actually be better for you, as you'll have a lot of plant-based options that are naturally gluten and wheat-free. As with any diet, you'll simply need to avoid the same products, such as whole wheat, bread, and baking products and other snacks or sauces that contain gluten or gluten-related products.

Question: Can I follow a plant-based diet if I have a lot of allergies?

Answer: Yes, and it's easier than you think. Because most foods are not processed, there is a benefit to eating whole, natural foods in place of packaged options. This may, in time, alleviate allergies in some people. If your allergy is specific to an additive or ingredient that is found in packaged food, it will most likely be avoided in a vegan diet. Allergies to certain fruits and vegetables, while possible, can simply entail avoiding them completely, whether it's a citrus fruit or a specific vegetable that you cannot consume.

Question: How can I eat and choose vegan foods at holiday and other family events or social engagements?

Answer: Guaranteed, there are usually vegan options available. If you have the option to find out in advance, arrange so that your preference for plant-based foods is an option. For more informal family gatherings, bring a plate or two of your own vegan creations, and you may be pleasantly surprised by how well-received it is. Many people who have never tried a vegan diet do not realize how many options there are for meal planning and taste. If you've lost any weight or appear healthier and leaner, people will take notice and attribute this to your vegan diet, which makes a significant impact.

Question: Do vegans live longer, and can we live longer without disease as the result of a plant-based diet?

Answer: There are some promising studies that claim vegans may outlive their meat-eating counterparts. There is also research that may indicate lower incidents of disease, including cancer, heart disease, and memory loss conditions often associated with aging and other dietary factors. Eliminating animal fats and products from your diet can cause you to feel more energetic as well, which can motivate you to keep active and lose weight if needed, or tone and gain a better fitness level overall.

Question: How do I get the most out of vegan eating? Is it more variety or should I focus on the nutrition levels instead?

Answer: A variety of foods is going to keep people interested in plant-based eating, though adding foods and balancing your dietary choices based on nutrient content and levels are also vital to a healthy and balanced lifestyle. When considering which foods are best for protein, calcium, fiber, and antioxidants, consider dark leafy greens as a top choice for covering all these nutrients. Choose "superfoods" as much as possible, such as chia seeds, avocado, and coconut. If you want to increase the nutrient power in your smoothies, add flax or hemp protein powder or crushed seeds to your drink before processing in the blender. This will ensure you get more than enough in just one serving.

Question: Is vegan safe for people of advanced age? Our kids also allowed to follow a plant-based diet? Are there any age limitations?

Answer: In short, no, there shouldn't be any limitations, as plant-based eating is safe for everyone of all dietary needs. Providing a vegan diet for kids is a healthy option, though it's best to check with a physician, just in case they require additional nutrients and/or supplements. This may be especially crucial for kids with chronic health conditions or may need certain types of nutrients more than others. For mature adults, the same applies. Check with your doctor first, then determine how to get any additional supplements and vitamins you might need. In general, the vegan diet is healthy and shouldn't cause any negative reaction, unless you're avoiding a lot of nutrients and narrowing down your own selection.

Question: How can I work around a soy allergy on a vegan diet?

Answer: Soy-based foods make up a significant part of the vegan diet, though they can be replaced with other protein-based alternatives, such as nut-based kinds of milk, seitan, and choosing vegetables high in iron, protein, and calcium. Now more than ever, there are plenty of options for vegans, including both soy and non-soy products.

Question: How successful is long-term weight loss on a plant-based diet?

Answer: It's successful because your body is consuming less fat, carbohydrates, and unnatural foods overall, making it easier to lose weight, digest, and metabolize better, and keep the weight off.

Question: How can I introduce other people to a vegan diet? Are there any suggestions?

Answer: Focus on the choices that a plant-based or vegan diet provides, instead of the restrictions (no meat, no dairy, etc.). Anyone new to a plant-based diet may be pleasantly surprised by how many options are available to them and how much more accommodating stores, restaurants, and markets are towards the vegan lifestyle. It is also a lifestyle about compassion and mindfulness, which takes into consideration all the foods chosen for their quality and animal-free status. Motivating people to start a vegan diet can be challenging because the first (and key) item most will ask is: What do I eat without meat? How can I have dairy and cheese on a vegan diet? Going vegan should be done gradually, over time, for some people who are resistant to change, but want to adapt to it over time.

Question: Is it easier to eliminate meat-based and dairy foods in stages, or jump into the vegan diet completely at once?

Answer: For most people, starting with small changes is ideal, and gradually losing and replacing animal products and foods with plant-based options is usually recommended. There are some people who are eager to "jump" into the vegan way of life, and they may naturally be good at adapting, or simply want to reap the awards sooner rather than later. This may cause some people to switch back to non-vegan eating if they don't prepare ahead, as they may become discouraged at some point. If you jump into a plant-based diet, be prepared for your body to react to the sudden changes, but also note that once you become adjusted, the rewards will definitely be worthwhile.

Question: When I choose a restaurant, how likely the staff to accommodate a vegan diet?

Answer: Most restaurants offer vegan foods and are exceptional at accommodating their customers. It's always best to check in advance just to be certain. When in doubt, always have a few vegan snacks handy, just in case there is a lack of plant-based food, though often, you'll be pleasantly surprised at how most places will offer vegan food options.

Description

How can a plant-based diet enable you to lose the excess weight you need and improve your health? Eating well and trying new recipes is a great way to motivate weight loss. One of the healthiest and most sustainable ways to eat well is by following a plant-based or vegan diet. In this book, you'll discover 50 delicious recipes, all of which are easy to prepare and are made from common ingredients you are already aware of. Contrary to many opinions, a vegan diet doesn't have to be expensive or considered a specialized diet, when there are limitless varieties of fruits, vegetables, grains, nuts, seeds, and many other non-dairy and meat-free options.

This book will provide a wide range of information and recipes to start you on a successful path to plant-based eating, including:

- The importance of plant-based eating for your body and health

- How adapting to a vegan diet is easier on your digestive system and weight loss

- The impact of eating processed foods and meat on weight gain and disease

- Focusing on simple, easy-to-make recipes that don't cost a fortune and can be made with just a handful of ingredients

- Getting rid of bad eating habits and replacing them with new, healthier practices.

- Choosing the best foods for your diet: keeping it healthy and vegan

- Focusing on plant-based proteins and nutrients

When you begin a new plant-based diet, you'll need a variety of tasty recipes to begin:

- Breakfast smoothies with all-natural ingredients

- Soups and salads that can be enjoyed as meals or side dishes

- Main dinner recipes easy to make

- Snacks and desserts

Starting a plant-based diet doesn't have to be difficult or challenging if you have the right foods and recipes to choose from. A vegan diet opens a new world of taste that isn't often discovered in a meat-based diet. There are also many ways to enjoy some of the most common fruits and vegetables in our local grocery stores, as well as exploring many other plant-based foods that are both convenient and delicious. Overall, the goal of a plant-based diet is to achieve optimum health and achieve a healthy weight, both of which become much more attainable with veganism. Losing weight is part of the process while gaining a better level of health and living ethically are also major advantages of the diet. Once you discover the limitless options there are in plant-based eating, it will only become more enjoyable and adventurous when it comes to exploring a wide range of foods. This book is your first step to reaching your goal of weight loss and a better way of eating, not just in the short-term, but as part of a lifestyle that will improve the quality of your overall well-being.

Vegan Meal Prep

Recipe Book with Delicious Low-Cost Recipes for Ready Meals and Tasty Snacks, Treat your Body with a Healthy and Balanced Diet

By Michael Garavaglia

form the information ultimately takes. This includes copied versions of the work both physical, digital and audio unless express consent of the Publisher is provided beforehand. Any additional rights reserved.

Furthermore, the information that can be found within the pages described forthwith shall be considered both accurate and truthful when it comes to the recounting of facts. As such, any use, correct or incorrect, of the provided information will render the Publisher free of responsibility as to the actions taken outside of their direct purview. Regardless, there are zero scenarios where the original author or the Publisher can be deemed liable in any fashion for any damages or hardships that may result from any of the information discussed herein.

Additionally, the information in the following pages is intended only for informational purposes and should thus be thought of as universal. As befitting its nature, it is presented without assurance regarding its prolonged validity or interim quality. Trademarks that are mentioned are done without written consent and can in no way be considered an endorsement from the trademark holder.

Table of Contents

Chapter 1: Introduction

Questions: Do I Need to Take Supplements on a Vegan Diet?

Chapter 1: Introduction

The Benefits of a Vegan Diet

When most people consider the option of a plant-based or vegan diet, they first weigh the advantages and disadvantages. There are often a lot of misconceptions and myths about the benefits of a plant-based diet, and some people fall prey to these ideas, without taking the time to try vegan meals and choose fresh, natural foods for their diet. The reality of most diets is the high reliance on processed and packaged foods, which provide little or no sustenance or nutrient value.

Are there any disadvantages to a vegan diet? Overall, there are only advantages, though there are a lot of challenges and adjustments to make along the way so that your body and lifestyle can become used to a new way of eating.

Characteristics of a Plant-Based Diet	Advantages	Challenges
Choosing more fresh and whole foods from the produce aisle or	Easy to locate in a store, and often full of options and variety. You'll	For people who are not generally in the habit of eating fresh fruits and vegetables,

section of the supermarket	find fruit and/or vegetable for every meal and occasion	this process will take some getting used to.
Lower calories and high nutrients	Lower chances of nutrient deficiency. The ability to satisfy all your body's nutrition needs with plant-based foods alone.	Learning to accept that a plant-based diet does not have to be void of protein and other nutrients, commonly (and falsely) believed to be in meat products only
More options for protein sources	Many plant-based foods contain significant amounts of protein, including nuts, seeds, soy, and dark greens.	Overcoming the myth of thinking there isn't enough protein outside of animal-based foods to sustain a healthy diet. Once you discover the variety of protein sources, and how all essential amino acids contained in protein can be obtained through plant-based foods, it will get easier.
Dairy products are animal-based and not included in a vegan diet	All the nutrients contained in dairy foods can	It can take a while to get used to non-dairy alternatives,

be found in plant-based foods, including dairy alternatives, such as soy and nut-based milk, butter, and yogurts	especially when baking or using soy or nut-based milk as a topping or ingredient. Fortunately, new and improved products are continuously available and can be purchased in nearly every regular grocery store.

Basics to Include in your Kitchen and Shopping List

Once you decide to try a plant-based diet, you'll want to become familiar with all the options available and how to design a shopping list that will work best for you. To begin your plant-based shopping list, focus on simple items that are easy to find in a grocery store. If you prefer specialty items, they may be available in local farmers' markets and natural food stores. Due to the increase in popularity in vegan diets, most, if not all grocery stores offer a wide range of plant-based foods that complete a full diet for the vegan lifestyle. Some of the following items are good for beginners to the plant-based way of eating and those who are more experienced with vegan shopping and meal preparation:

Tofu

It may not be the first choice that comes to mind, or it might be a source of hesitation and avoidance if you haven't tried tofu before. Fortunately, tofu is a well-liked food for vegans and meat-eaters alike, for how easily it fits into many types of cuisine, from miso soup to pad thai, and a variety of stir-fries, bakes, and desserts. Try both firm and soft (silken) tofu to gain a better idea of the benefits for both. Firm versions of tofu are best for baking, marinating for stir-fries and soups. Soft or silken tofu is ideal for creating puddings or sauces. Include tofu on your shopping list often.

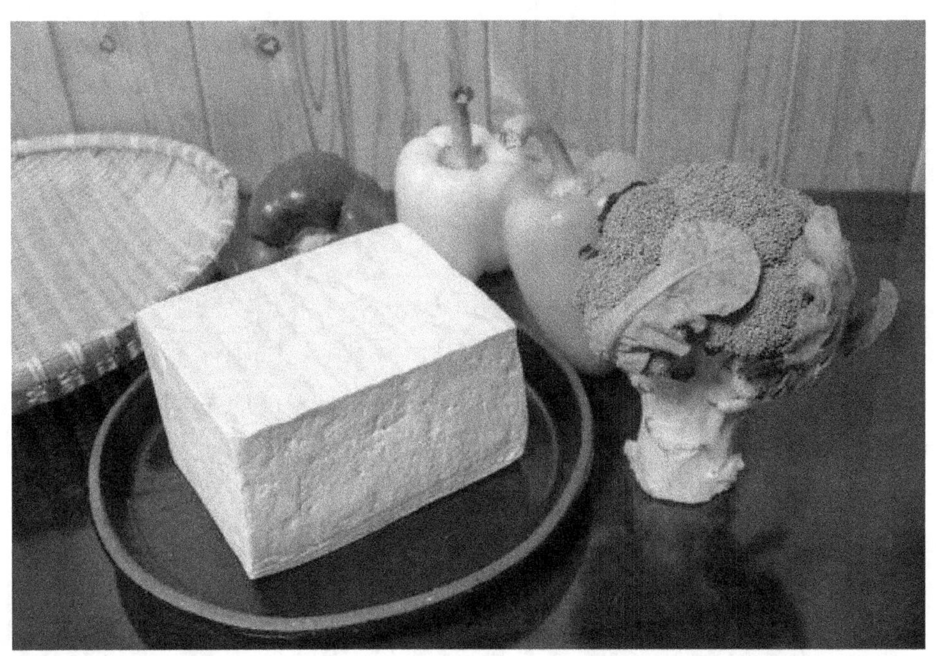

Tempeh

Also, a soy-based food, tempeh has a more firm texture that is more like "meat" and is often successfully used as a meat substitute for this reason. Tempeh is excellent for marinating for pasta, stir-fries, and salads.

Dark Green Vegetables

Choose at least one dark green vegetable each week during your grocery shopping. Kale, arugula, cabbage, parsley, spinach, and broccoli are all great examples. Anyone of these vegetables can be added to stews, soups or sliced and stirred into a skillet meal or salad. Dark leafy greens and green vegetables, in general, are some of the most nutrient-rich foods on the planet and should definitely remain on your shopping list each week.

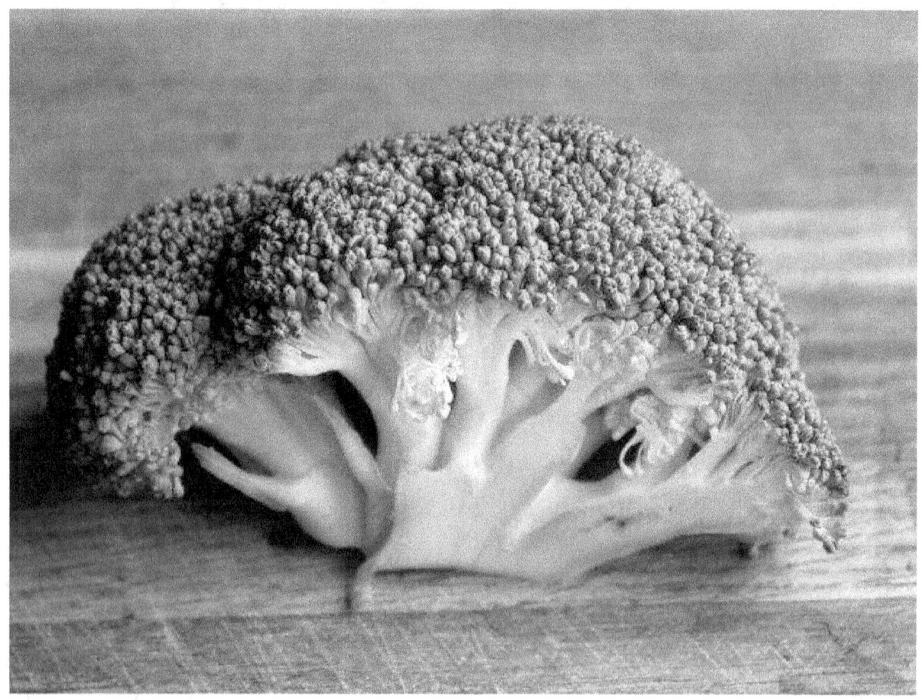

Quinoa

One of the most nutritious grains to select, quinoa combines a number of vitamins, protein, and minerals into one grain. It's a great substitute for rice and other grains often added as a side dish or as a soup or salad ingredient. Other options for grains to consider include barley, wild rice, brown rice, oats, and millet.

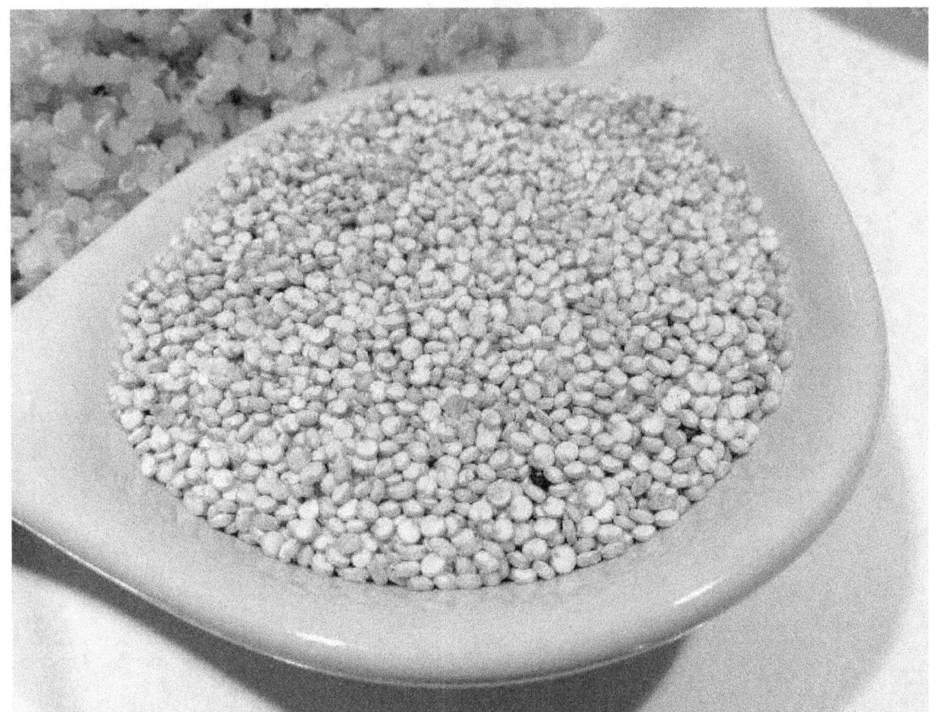

Fresh Fruits

Nature's source of sweetness and a perfect snack, choose a few different fruits each week, or as many as you can. Apples, oranges, kiwi, berries (any variety), pineapple, peaches, and mangoes are all excellent options. Avocado is also a fruit that is often mistaken as a vegetable and used in a few recipes included in this book.

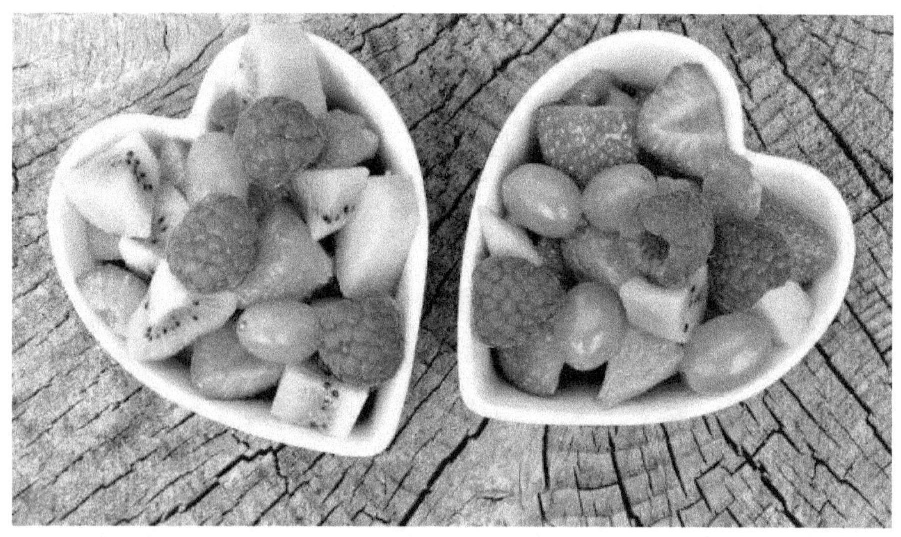

Non-Dairy Options

Once you begin exploring the vegan world of cooking and baking, you'll want to become familiar with dairy alternatives, including coconut, soy, and nut-based milk, yogurt, and butter. Vegan cheese is often soy or vegetable-based. Other dairy alternatives include sour cream, cream cheese and whipping cream. Coconut based products tend to be thick and easily resemble cream or whole dairy milk as a suitable replacement in recipes. Soy and almond milk are the most popular and available in most grocery stores.

Oats

Consider this item as a staple in your diet, especially if you need energy in the morning and wish to create some creative breakfast options included in the recipe section of this book. Oats are very high in nutrients and work well with many ingredients to create a number of tasty breakfast meals.

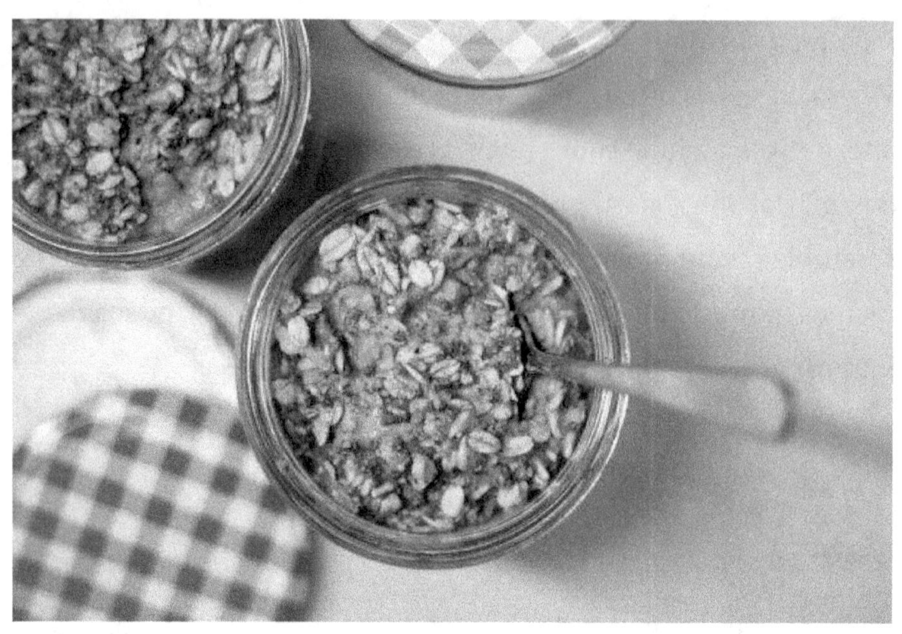

Nuts and Seeds

Almonds, cashews, pistachios, walnuts, pecans, and peanuts are all high in protein and fiber. Choose at least one per week as a snack option or ingredients in a recipe of your choice. Chia, hemp, and flax seeds are also fantastic for ensuring you get the antioxidants and fiber you need on a daily basis. These superfoods are often available in bulk stores and always in grocery stores.

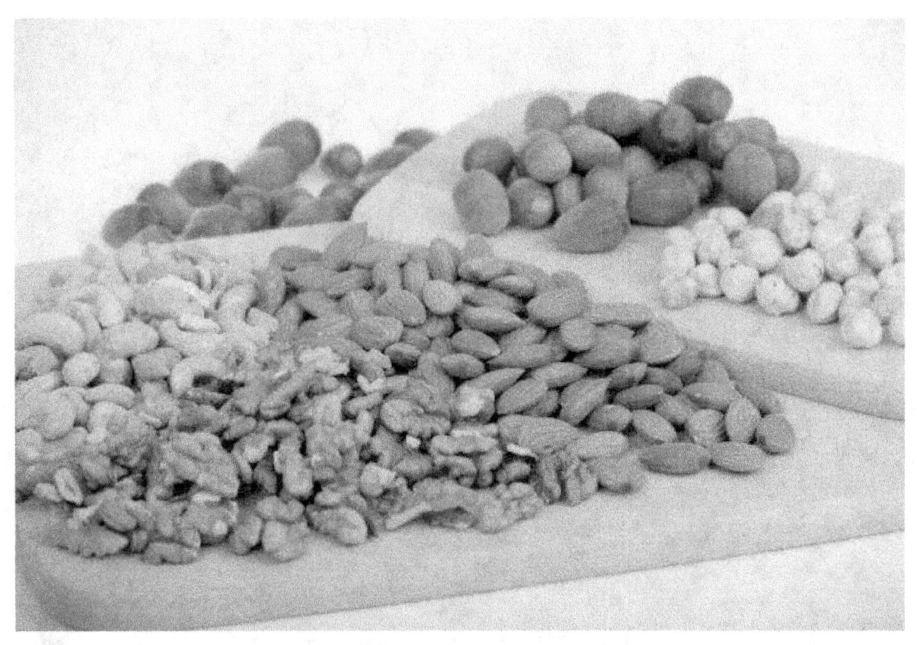

Spices and Herbs

Add as many spices and herbs as you can, so that you can create your pantry and have the main options available for any dish you enjoy. Common spices include black pepper, salt, chili powder, turmeric, cinnamon, cardamom, paprika, nutmeg, curry, and cloves. Check the ingredient lists of the recipes you wish to try, and create a list based on the items you need. Once you build your pantry, it will become easier as you only have to replace or top up on certain items. Herbs are another great way to flavor food and include rosemary, rosehip, masala chai, and tarragon.

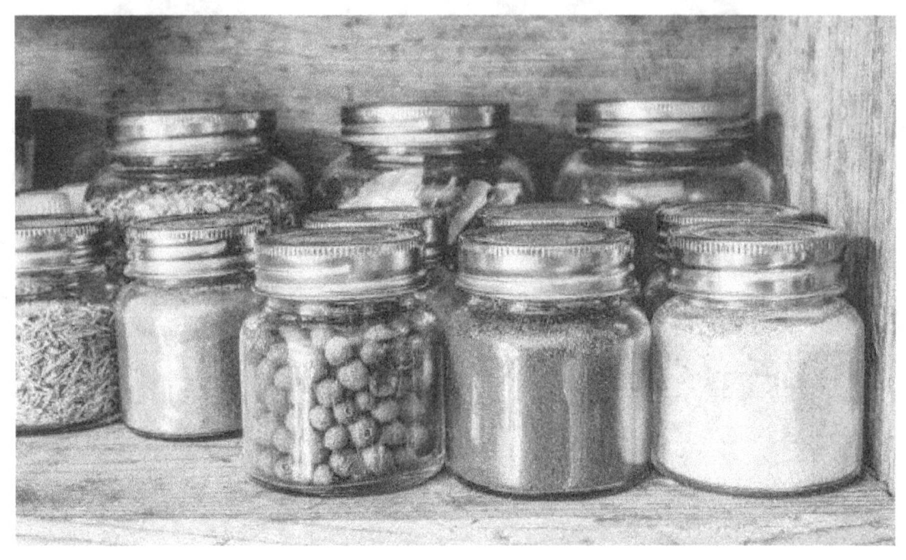

Other foods to include on your shopping trip? Consider the outer sections of the grocery store where most of the fresh foods are located, including the produce section. There are many new and interesting healthy snacks, smoothies, and meal preparation ideas, some of which are delicious and healthy, though some contain artificial ingredients. Some good options to consider include the following:

- Vegan condiments: not all of these products are created equal, and some are more artificially flavored than others.

In small amounts, most vegan sauces and condiments are acceptable.

- Dried fruits are a great snack option. Be sure to choose sun-dried fruits only, or avoid unnecessary additives.

- Frozen fruits and vegetables: These are a good option when fresh is not an option.

- Whole wheat, and gluten-free flour. Baking goods and ingredients, in general, are important to have on hand. If in doubt, always make sure you have the following three ingredients at home for a variety of dishes: flour, baking soda, and baking powder. Vanilla extract is another good item to have on hand for baking and creating desserts.

Always read the ingredients and labels for all the foods you buy, and if possible, skip the packaged foods as much as possible and make fresh and natural options the main goal. Filling your cart with more raw fruits and vegetables is ideal and should take a priority over dried or processed foods.

Chapter 2: Recipes for Vegan Breakfasts and Smoothies

Breakfast Recipes

There are many great plant-based, breakfast recipes that can be prepared quickly in the morning, or prepared the night before, for an easy, enjoyable, and effortless meal the next day. The first meal of the day can be a task, especially if the morning is the busiest time of the day. Most people grab a banana or energy bar, though sometimes breakfast can take an unhealthy turn with sugary cereals and artificially flavored meal replacements. The recipes below provide options for eating quickly, or during occasions when you can indulge in a late brunch with family and friends.

Crepes

Instead of heavy pancakes and sugary crepes, there are alternative ways to create tasty, even decadent crepes and fillings. Crepes are easy to make with a light batter that combines tapioca and almond flour with coconut milk. These three ingredients will ensure a light and thin crepe that can be used as a base for many filling and topping options.

- 1 cup of tapioca flour

- 1 cup of almond flour
- 2 teaspoons of coconut flour (optional)
- 1 cup of coconut milk
- 1 teaspoon of vanilla extract
- Olive oil to heat the skillet

In a medium or large bowl, combine the two flours (plus the coconut flour, if including this as an option), mix thoroughly. Gently pour in the coconut milk and vanilla extract and whisk at the same time with the other hand, ensuring a gentle mix where there are no lumps or inconsistencies in the blending of the ingredients. If necessary, use an electric mixer for a smooth result, or simply whisk thoroughly until ready. Heat a skillet on medium, pour a five or six-inch disk of thin batter and gently fry for about two minutes on each side, or until lightly golden. Remove and place on a plate and add your choice of filling.

There are many filling and topping ideas for a crepe. Consider some of the following combinations:

- Fill a crepe with one mashed banana and almond butter, roll and sprinkle with cocoa powder.
- Add fresh strawberries, blueberries, raspberries and/or blackberries and top with coconut whipped cream.

- Fill with sliced mango or peach, and drizzle coconut milk or cream, and top with icing sugar.

- Add melted dark chocolate, peanut butter, and a banana (optional) and top with cocoa powder.

- In a bowl, mash a banana with some coconut or almond milk, and fill the crepe with this mix and a handful of crushed almonds, pistachios and/or peanuts. Top with cinnamon

- Two tablespoons of pumpkin puree with pumpkin spices and a dollop of coconut whipping cream or vanilla tofu pudding.

- If you want to keep it simple, serve plain with a drizzle of maple syrup

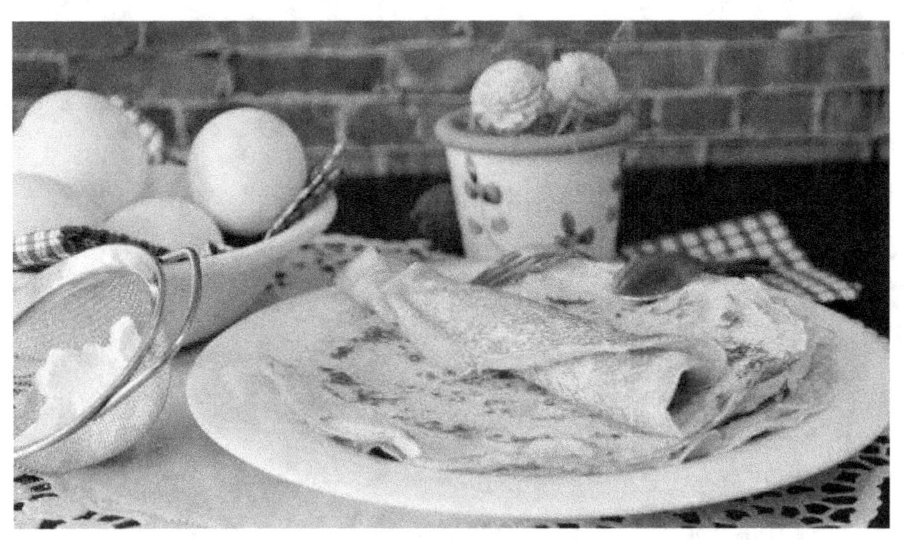

Chocolate Crepes

If you want a twist on the simple version of the crepe recipe,
consider adding a little cocoa powder for a chocolate version:

- 1 cup of tapioca flour
- 1 cup of almond flour
- 1 cup of coconut milk
- 1 teaspoon of vanilla extract
- 2 tablespoons of cocoa powder
- Olive oil to heat the skillet

Prepare the skillet as the recipe above. In a large bowl, combine
the two flours and cocoa powder and mix thoroughly, then
slowly pour in the coconut milk and vanilla extract to gradually
blend smoothly. Pour the mixture (five or six-inch diameter is
recommended) and fry on both sides evenly for about two or
three minutes. Serve on a plate and top with coconut whipping
cream and any combination of toppings and/or fillings desired.

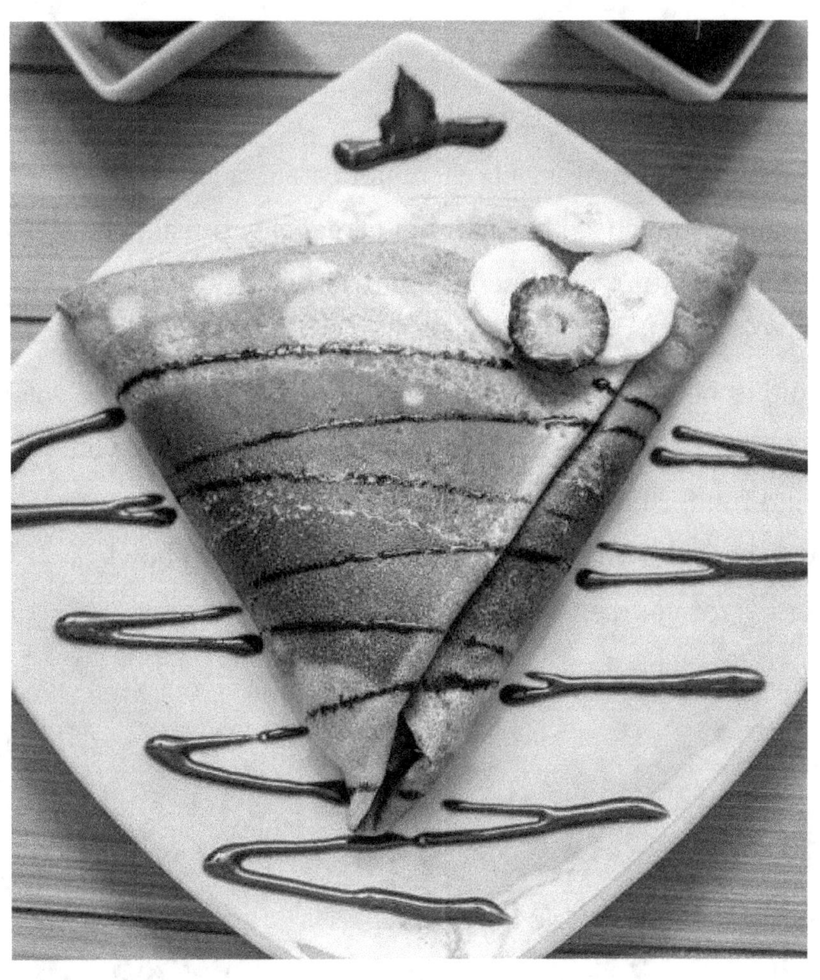

Hot Cereal

During the colder months, a bowl of hot cereal is ideal. The most popular and widely used base for hot cereal is oatmeal, which provides a good source of fiber and nutrients. Grains, like oatmeal, tend to digest slowly, which helps you feel fuller longer and avoid unnecessary hunger pangs. A bowl of oatmeal is also a deeply satisfying meal in taste and texture that will keep you warm and full for hours. There are many options and flavor themes to consider when creating your own oatmeal bowl, whether it's for yourself only or several servings.

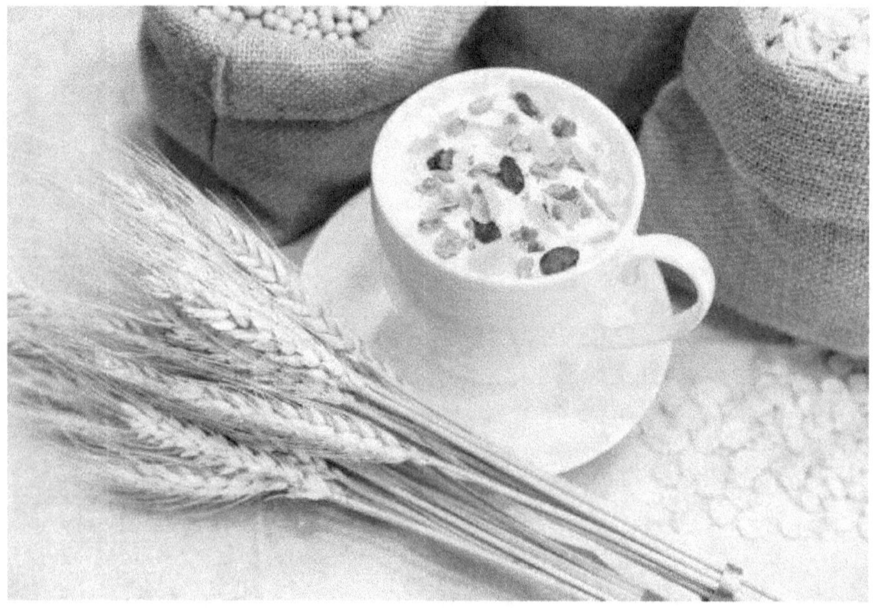

Apple Cinnamon Oatmeal

If you have a few apples sitting in the crisper of your refrigerator, they will make a great addition to your oatmeal, while adding some fiber and vitamins. Cinnamon is a tasty spice that complements the taste of apple. Other ingredients included in this recipe increase the nutrient content to make this a tasty meal to enjoy.

- 2 cups of rolled oats
- 3 cups of water
- 1 cup of almond milk
- 1 medium or 2 small apples, peeled, cored, and sliced
- 2 tablespoons of cinnamon
- 1 tablespoon of chia seeds
- 1 tablespoon of hemp seeds
- 2 tablespoons of maple syrup, raw sugar, or a low carb sweetener
- ½ cup of almond milk

In a large cooking pot, pour the water and almond milk and heat on medium-high to bring to a boil. Slowly pour in the oats and continue to stir evenly, ensuring all of the oats mixtures. Stir in the chia seeds and hemp seeds and continue to mix, while reducing the heat to a medium-low setting. On a small cutting board, peel and core the apples, then cut into small cubes or slices and add to the oatmeal, stirring them in evenly. Cover and cook on low for about 12-15 minutes more, or until all the apples are softened. Add in the cinnamon and stir gently, then pour into bowls and serve. This recipe makes approximately 4-6 servings. Top with coconut cream or almond milk and sprinkle extra cinnamon or raw sugar on top.

There are a few variations to consider for this recipe:

- Substitute 2-3 tablespoons of apple sauce in place of apples, for a smoother texture

- Apple butter is another option to add for a slightly different texture and taste, either with apples or in addition to them.

Maple Syrup Oatmeal

If you enjoy the taste of maple, this recipe is not only simple but delicious and will take only three ingredients to prepare.

- 2 cups of rolled oats
- 3 cups of water
- 1 cup of almond milk
- 2 tablespoons of maple syrup

Bring the water and milk to a bowl in one cooking pot, then pour in the oats and stir, cooking for at least 5-6 minutes, then reduce heat to medium and pour in the maple syrup, gently mixing into the oats. If desired, add an extra tablespoon of syrup or some raw sugar to enhance the sweetness. Remove from heat and serve in bowls.

Power Oatmeal Breakfast

If you're focused on getting a boost of protein and nutrients from your morning bowl of oatmeal, this is an ideal combination to try. This involves a medley of both nuts and seeds and a dash of flavor.

- 1 ½ cups of rolled oats
- ½ cup of chia seeds
- ¼ cup of slivered almonds
- 2 tablespoons of hemp seeds
- 1 tablespoon of crushed flax seeds
- 1 tablespoon of soy vanilla protein powder or one tablespoon of tahini (softened at room temperature)
- 2 tablespoons of maple syrup or raw sugar (or low carb sweetener)
- 1 ½ cups of water
- 1 ½ cups of almond or hemp milk

Pour the water and milk into a large cooking pot and bring to a boil. In a large bowl, combine the oats, hemp seeds, flax seeds, almonds, and vanilla protein powder. Mix thoroughly and pour into the boiling water and milk, gently stirring. Add in the tahini (if used in place of the protein powder), followed by the maple syrup, sugar, or sweetener. Continue to cook on medium heat for another 14-15 minutes until all seeds and oats are softened, which may take up to 20 minutes. Remove from heat and serve topped with cinnamon, cocoa, and/or almond milk.

If you want a thicker result for any of the above oatmeal recipes, consider using more milk and less water, or use coconut milk in place of almond or hemp milk as an option.

Overnight Oats

Oats, chia seeds, hemp, and flax seeds are just some excellent high-nutrient examples of what you can include in a custom-made mix of ingredients in a jar or bowl of overnight oats. The greatest advantage of this recipe? It only takes a few minutes to prepare the night before, and requires no cooking, boiling or additional preparation the next morning to enjoy. There are also many variations on flavor and ingredients, which make this a dish you can experiment with by adding or changing the types of layers you wish to combine.

Each overnight oatmeal recipe consists of non-dairy milk, oats, and toppings. The type of milk you choose may include rice, soy, hemp, almond, cashew, or oat milk. There are a growing number of nut-based milk becoming available in natural food stores, as well as your local grocery store, making them a convenience. They tend to be comparable in price to the dairy version, and some cartons can be stored in the pantry as long as they are sealed and refrigerated once opened. Coconut milk is a good option of rich, creamy-textured recipes, while almond, cashew, and other nut milk are good for peanut butter and similar flavors, including those combined with cocoa or chocolate.

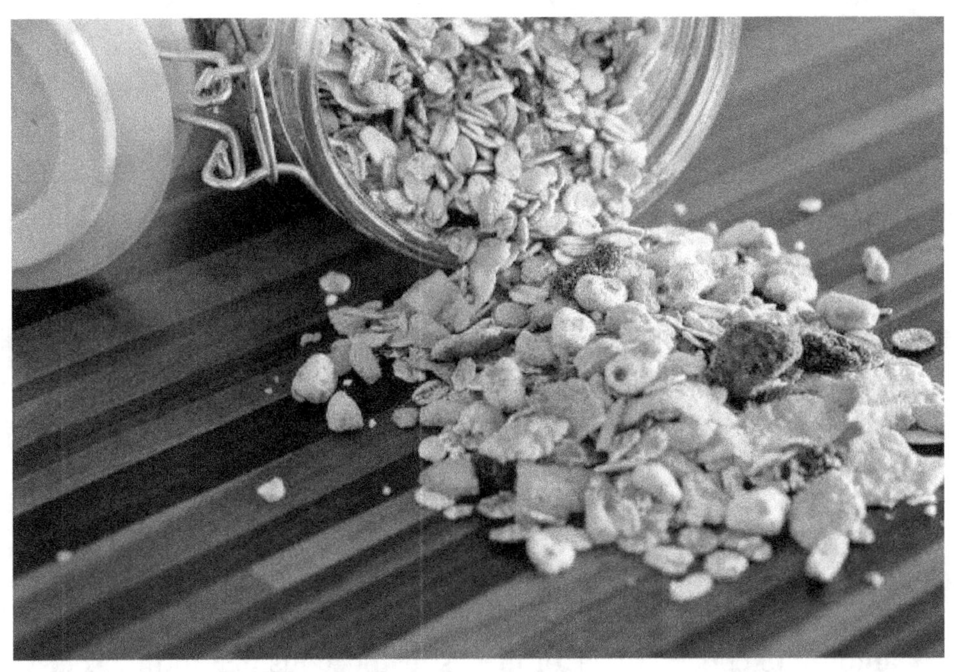

Peanut Butter Chocolate Overnight Oats

This recipe is excellent for chocolate and peanut butter fans and has the potential to provide a heaping portion of healthy fats and protein in one serving. The best type of milk to use for this recipe is almond, cashew or nut milk, though hemp milk is another option that works well with this blend of flavor. The type of chocolate used should be raw cocoa or a dark variety of chocolate without dairy. Baker's chocolate offers this option, which can be melted on low heat or microwaved, before combining with other ingredients. To double or increase the amount of chocolate flavor in this recipe, consider adding cocoa or chocolate-flavored nut-based milk. Some varieties of almond milk offer a chocolate version of this drink.

- 2 tablespoons of cocoa powder or the equivalent melted the dark chocolate
- 2 tablespoons of raw sugar, low carb sweetener or maple syrup
- 2 tablespoons of peanut butter, softened at room temperature
- 1 cup of oats
- 1 cup of milk (almond, cashew, hazelnut, or hemp milk)

In a medium-sized jar, combine the milk with the oats, then stir in the cocoa powder or chocolate (melted), mixing gently to combine the ingredients. Add in the peanut butter and sweetener and continue to stir. As an option, add in chocolate chips and/or crushed peanuts for texture.

Blueberry Overnight Oatmeal

Naturally sweet, blueberries tend to pair well with oatmeal and milk as a great way to add a rich flavor and added sweetness, without any artificial flavors. The best option for blueberries is fresh, though frozen (and thawed) is also a good alternative. If you decide to add dried blueberries, they will "plump" overnight. Coconut milk is a good option for a creamier, dessert-like texture, though any type of milk or non-dairy yogurt will work perfectly in this recipe.

- 1 cup of fresh blueberries
- 1 cup of rolled oats
- 1 ½ cups of coconut milk, or
- ½ cup of coconut or non-dairy yogurt and 1 cup of non-dairy milk
- 2 teaspoons of raw sugar, maple syrup or low carb sweetener

Combine all ingredients except for the blueberries in a medium jar. Add the oats, milk (and optional yogurt), and sweetener first, stirring together, then fold in the blueberries until well combined and refrigerate overnight. For added protein and nutrients, add in a tablespoon of chia seeds or crushed almonds.

Banana and Strawberry Overnight Oatmeal

Like a smoothie, this oatmeal treat combines well with banana and strawberries and tastes like a dessert. Bananas can be added to this recipe in a few different ways: by slicing into disks, and gently mixing or folding into the ingredients, along with the strawberries, or mashed and blended with the milk and oats first, or mashed and added at the end, either with the berries or separately. If you have an overripe banana, it can be used for this recipe easily and blended with the milk in a food processor, then mixed with the oats and strawberries.

- 1 ripe banana
- 1 ½ cups of soy, almond or another non-dairy milk
- 2 teaspoons of sweetener
- 4-5 large fresh, medium strawberries, stems removed and sliced
- 1 cup of rolled oats

In a medium jar, combine the oats and milk and stir in the sweetener. Before adding the milk, the banana can be processed together in a blender with the milk, then combined with the oats and sweetener, or simply add the chopped slices of the strawberries and bananas together and fold into the mixed oats. Drizzle with maple syrup or sprinkle with raw sugar, if desired.

Coconut Overnight Oatmeal

This recipe focuses on the rich, pleasant taste of coconut, by blending a few layers: coconut milk, cream, and shredded or dried coconut flakes.

- I cup of rolled oats
- 1 ½ cups of coconut milk
- ¼ cups of shredded coconut
- 1 tablespoon of coconut cream
- 1 tablespoon of raw or coconut sugar

Combine and stir the oats, coconut milk, cream, and sugar together, then add in ½ of the shredded coconut and fold into the oatmeal before chilling overnight. Serve with lightly toasted or raw shredded coconut on top.

Almond Delight Overnight Oatmeal

Almond butter, extract and sliced nuts are combined to create a rich and creamy dessert-like version of overnight oats. Add almond cream for a slightly thicker texture (your grocery store may provide non-dairy creamers which can be added as well).

- ½ cup of almond butter
- 1 teaspoon almond extract
- ½ cup of sliced or slivered almonds
- 1 cup of oats
- 1 ½ cups of almond milk
- 2 teaspoons maple syrup of natural sweetener

In a bowl, combine the almond butter and oats, then stir in the almond extract and sweetener. Transfer to a medium jar and pour in with the almond milk. Once gently mixed, fold in the sliced or slivered almonds.

Smoothies

Smoothies are convenient, easy, and fast to create and enjoy if you are often rushed and out of time to make a full meal. Not only are smoothies an excellent source of nutrients, but they can also replace a meal any time of day, and sustain your appetite until the next meal. Most smoothies only require three or four ingredients, with some variations and options available. The combinations of ingredients and flavors are limitless, as there are many ideas to explore, depending on your own personal tastes. Smoothies can often be prepared on the go with just a few items left in your refrigerator and/or cupboard.

Cocoa and Almond Butter Smoothie

A refreshing yet rich-tasting smoothie, this drink will give you the energy needed to begin your day. Raw cocoa is recommended, though any dark chocolate will work for this recipe. Almond butter should be kept at room temperature until soft enough to blend with the cocoa and milk.

- 3 tablespoons of raw cocoa powder or melted dark chocolate
- ½ cup of almond butter
- 2 cups of almond milk

- 2 teaspoons of maple syrup or low carb sweetener

Combine all items in a blender and pulse for 30 seconds, or until smooth. This recipe creates at least one serving.

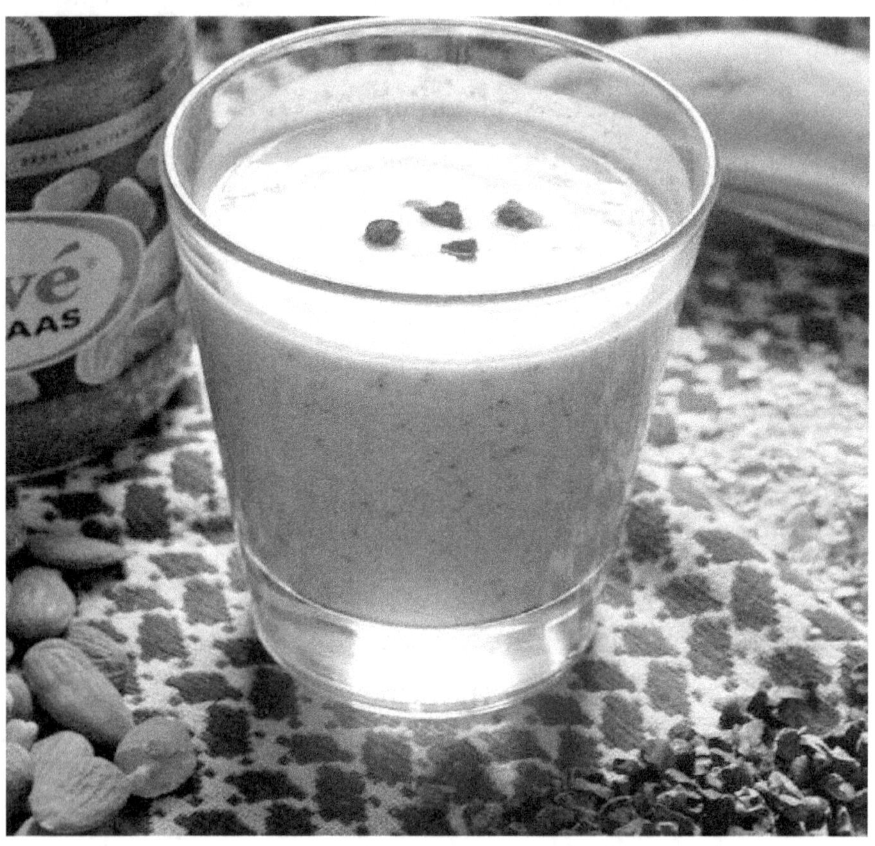

Banana, Coconut and Avocado Smoothie

If you need a lot of fiber, healthy fats, and protein in one serving, this is an excellent smoothie option. Avocadoes used for this drink should be very ripe, though not overripe, so they can be blended easily with the other ingredients. The banana should be ripe enough to blend with ease as well.

- 1 ripe banana
- 1 ripe avocado (medium)
- 2 ½ cups of coconut milk
- 1 teaspoon of shredded coconut or coconut cream

Combine all ingredients in the blender and pulse until smooth. If the result is too thick, add another ½ cup of milk, then blend for another 15-20 seconds, until ready to serve.

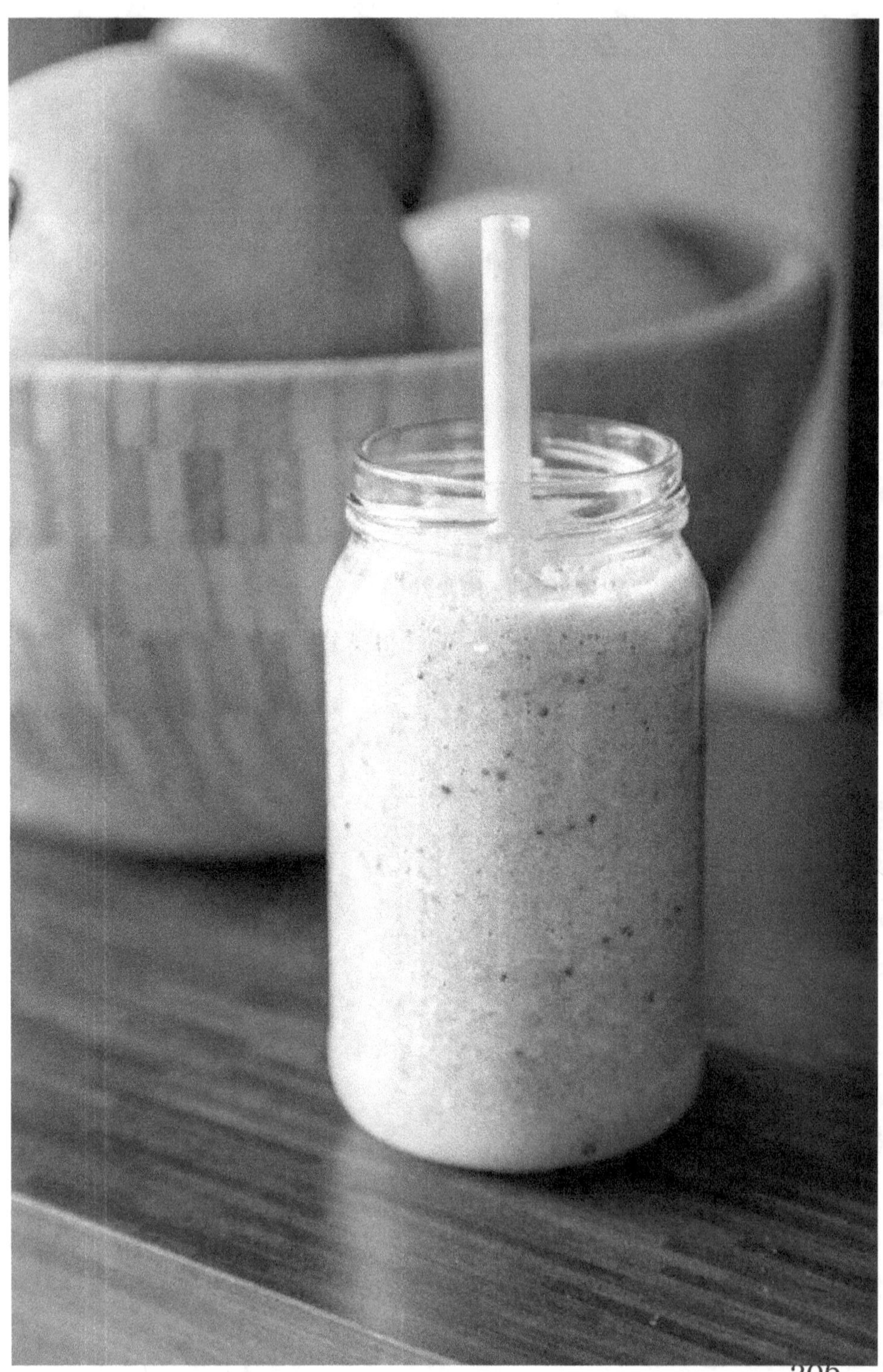

Cherry and Blueberry Smoothie

The antioxidant power of berries includes a good dose of prevention against a lot of disease and chronic ailments. Cherries and blueberries both tend to be the sweetest berries, and especially in combination, they can replace the need for a sweetener. Cherries are high in alkaline, which helps reduce inflammation while blueberries contain high amounts of vitamin C.

- ½ cup of pitted cherries
- ½ cup of blueberries
- ½ a banana
- 2 cups of almond milk

Combine all ingredients into the blender and mix for a minimum of 60 seconds. The berries can be either fresh or frozen. If preferred, the banana can be omitted completely and replaced with 1-2 tablespoons of vanilla soy protein powder.

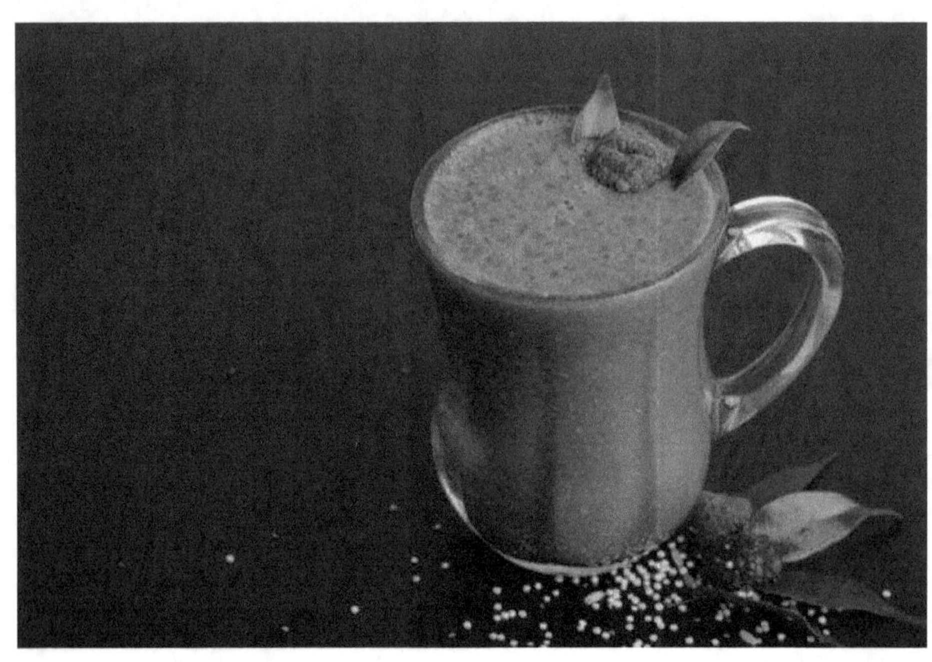

Pumpkin Spice and Banana Smoothie

This recipe will replace a meal any time of day, and give you the potassium, fiber, and vitamins you need. Fresh pumpkin isn't usually in season, which makes pureed canned pumpkin the best option most of the time. Just one small can of pumpkin is enough, or you can add half of a small or large can, depending on how much pumpkin flavor you want.

- 1 ripe banana
- 1 small can of pureed pumpkin (or half a large can)
- 1 teaspoon of cinnamon
- 1 teaspoon of nutmeg
- ½ teaspoon of cloves
- 2 teaspoons of maple syrup or raw sugar
- 2 cups of almond milk

Combine the banana, pumpkin puree, and milk in the blender first and pulse for 45 seconds or slightly longer, until smooth. Add in the spices and sweetener and mix for another 30-45 seconds. Add in some ice cubes to crush and chill the drink or enjoy it as is. This recipe makes about 2-3 servings.

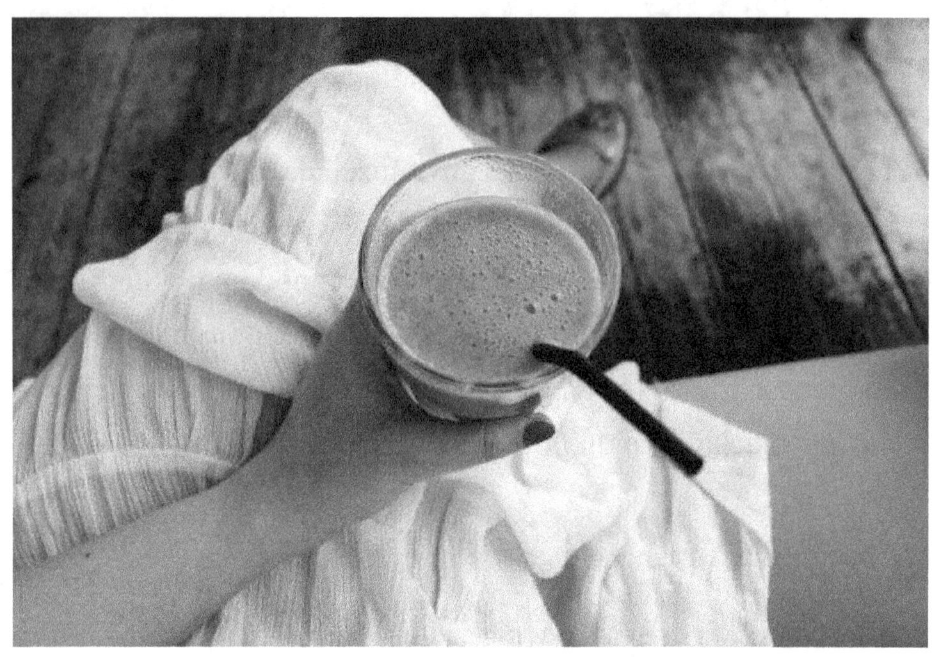

Peanut Butter and Coconut Smoothie

The combination of natural peanut butter and coconut milk provides the ultimate combination of healthy fats all in one smoothie. Coconut milk is thicker than nut-based milk and may need some added almond or soymilk to help this smoothie blend well.

- ½ cups of peanut butter (smooth, unsalted, and unsweetened)
- 1 cup of coconut milk
- ½ cup of almond or soymilk
- 2 tablespoons of shredded coconut
- 2 tablespoons of raw sugar or maple syrup
- 1 teaspoon of almond extract

Combine the soymilk or almond milk and coconut milk together in a blender, then add in the peanut butter and pulse for 60 seconds. Add in the sweetener, almond extract, and shredded coconut, and continue to blend until smooth. This drink provides about 2-3 servings.

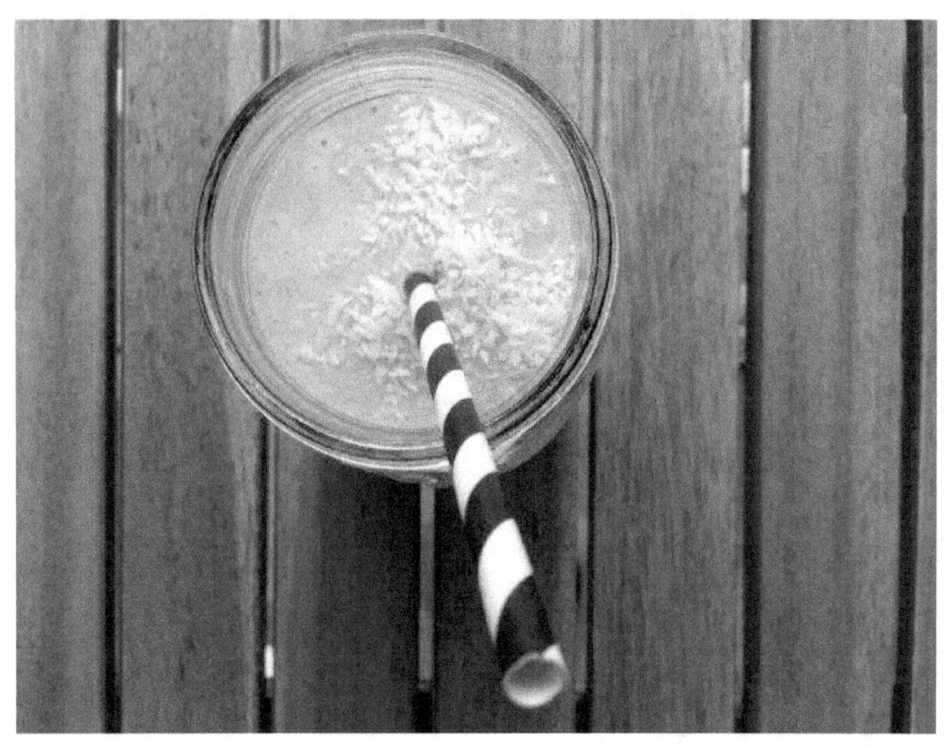

Chapter 3: Snacks and Side Dish Recipes

Plant-based snacks and light meals don't have to be bland or dull. In fact, there are many options to flavor vegetables to create delicious snacks whether it's with a bit of spice or a marinated sauce or curry. Many vegetables have great flavor on their own, with just the right amount of steaming, baking, or frying, sometimes with very minimal spice and herbs. This chapter offers a collection of vegan recipes that will give you quick options on the go or as a delicious side or light meal at home

Plant-Based Snacks

Chips, chocolate bars and other sugary or high-sodium snacks can be tempting, and they are often located in the most inconvenient (or convenient) spots in the supermarket and corner stores. It can be too easy to grab a quick snack from this aisle on the go, though it can become habit-forming and cause a regular indulgence of unhealthy eating. Designing snacks that work best for a plant-based diet means getting more out of your meal in terms of nutrition and taste. Healthier, nutrient-rich snacks also fill you quickly and satisfy your hunger, which reduces the chances of overeating.

Garlic Roasted Chickpeas

This snack is easily prepared with just a few ingredients. A spare can of chickpeas in the pantry and a few spices can create a wonderful, protein-rich snack within just 25-30 minutes of preparation and baking in the oven. Garlic powder is usually bought for soups and stews and works well to add a strong flavor to the otherwise mild, yet pleasant taste of chickpeas.

- 1 can of chickpeas drained and rinsed
- 2 tablespoons of garlic powder
- 1 teaspoon of sea salt
- 1 teaspoon of black pepper
- ¼ cup of olive oil

In a large bowl, toss the drained chickpeas and oil, then sprinkle with garlic, salt, and black pepper mix, tossing the chickpeas gently, until they are all evenly coated. Heat the oven to 350 degrees and line a baking sheet with parchment paper. Spread the chickpeas across the sheet, and place in the preheated oven. Bake for approximately 20-25 minutes, or until slightly brown.

Keep a close eye on the beans between 20-25 minutes, to ensure they do not overcook or burn. Remove from heat, cool, then serve.

Curry Roasted Chickpeas

A twist on the traditional Chana masala meal, which involves stewing chickpeas in a curry, this recipe simply adds the curry powder into a bowl the lightly olive oil-coated chickpeas and bakes in approximately 20 minutes. Garam masala and chili powder can also be added to enhance the curry flavor.

- 1 can of chickpeas, drained and rinsed
- 2 tablespoons of curry powder
- ¼ cups of olive oil
- 1 teaspoon of garam masala
- 1 teaspoon of chili powder (optional)
- Dash of sea salt
- Dash of black pepper

Combine the spices together in a small bowl and set aside. In a large bowl, toss in the chickpeas and coat evenly, then add in the spices and fold gently to ensure all beans are coated. Transfer the chickpeas to a baking sheet and bake for 20-25 minutes. Remove from the oven, cool, then serve.

Both chickpea recipes above can be stored at room temperature for up to one week in a resealable container and make an excellent snack on the go. Just one half of a cup of roasted chickpeas are a great way to get the protein and fiber you need quickly and especially in between meals. They also make an excellent topping on salads as well.

Spicy Garlic Kale Chips

Kale is a superfood that provides many antioxidants, iron, magnesium, calcium, and fiber to your diet. While kale has a bitter taste in its raw form, it blends well in many dishes, and can easily be baked into tasty chips as a healthy snack. This recipe blends garlic powder and chili pepper to create spicy and flavorful chips for any occasion. These are easy to make and only take about 10 minutes to bake in a conventional oven. Just one bunch of kale can make several baking sheets covered in chips, and more. In stores, kale chips tend to be expensive, though they can be made with just a few ingredients within 15-20 minutes.

- 1 bunch of raw kale leaves (stems removed, sliced in one or two-inch pieces)
- 2 tablespoons of garlic powder
- 1 teaspoon of chili powder
- Dash of sea salt
- Olive oil to coat kale

Heat the oven to 350 degrees and prepare a baking sheet lined with paper. Wash and thoroughly drain the kale and remove the stems. Slice the leaves into bite-sized pieces (up to two inches in diameter) and set in a large bowl. Pour 1/8 cups of olive oil into a small bowl and using your fingers, lightly coat each slice of kale and place on the baking sheet. In another bowl, mix the garlic powder, sea salt, and chili pepper and sprinkle over each of the kale chips. Bake in the oven for approximately 8-10 minutes, until slightly crispy, then remove from heat, cool slightly, and enjoy. Kale chips can be stored at room temperature for up to one week, in a sealable container.

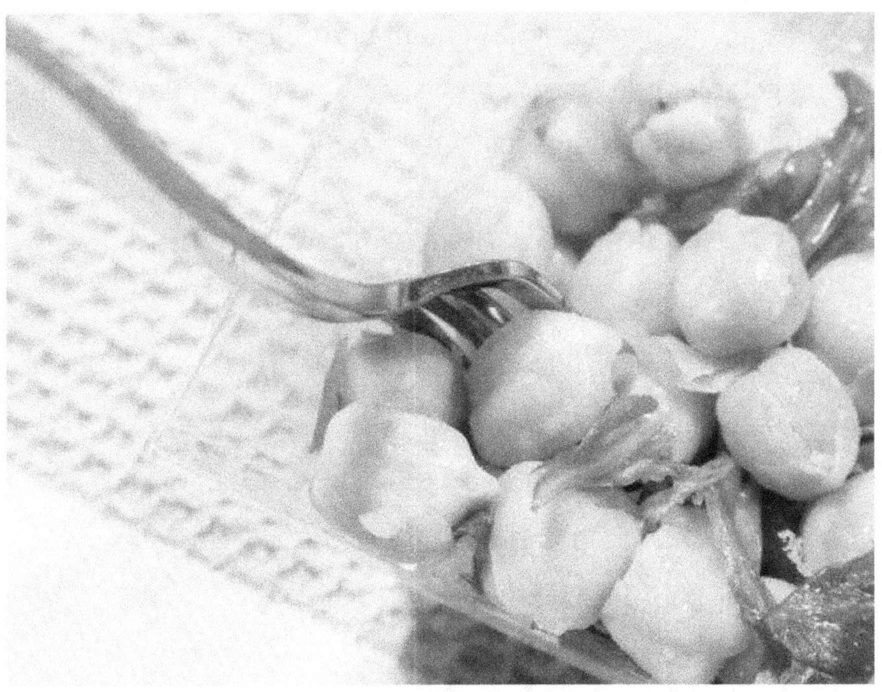

Side Dishes

Fried Curried Cabbage

A quick, tasty side dish or a light meal, curried cabbage is easier to make than you may think. Cabbage contains a wealth of nutrients, including vitamin C and fiber. It blends well with other vegetables and spices and becomes mellow in flavor when cooked. This dish requires just a few ingredients in a skillet to get started.

- 2 cups of shredded cabbage
- ½ small onion, diced
- 2 tablespoons of curry powder
- ½ teaspoon of turmeric
- 1 teaspoon of chili powder
- ½ teaspoon garlic powder
- 1 teaspoon of black pepper
- 1 teaspoon of sea salt
- 2 tablespoons of olive oil

In a medium to a large skillet, add in the olive oil and heat on medium. Add in the diced onion, curry powder, turmeric, chili powder, garlic powder, black pepper, and sea salt. Sauté for about 5-6 minutes, then toss in the shredded cabbage and reduce heat to medium-low, continuing to cook until all cabbage is gently coated in oil and curry. Cabbage should be tender, though slightly crunchy. Remove from heat and serve on rice or on a plate as a side or main dish.

**Mashed Yams**

This recipe is just like mashed potatoes and takes about the same time frame to prepare. Choose yams that are small or medium in size. Skins can be left on or peeled off before adding. Garlic cloves can be combined with the yams to create a stronger taste.

- 4-5 yams, washed and scrubbed (peeled or skins left on)
- 2 cloves of garlic (optional)
- 1 teaspoon of black pepper
- 6 cups of water
- Dash of sea salt
- 2 tablespoons vegan butter
- 1 cup of soymilk (plain, unsweetened)

In a large cooking pot, pour in the water and add the sea salt. Slice the yams into small, one or two-inch cubes or pieces and add to the water. Bring to a boil, then reduce heat and cook on medium until yams are soft. If desired, add the cloves 9f garlic to the yams at the same time, cooking them together. Continue to cook on medium until the yams and garlic are tender, then drain in a colander and pour into a large bowl. Mash together with vegan butter, one cup of soymilk and a dash of sea salt and black pepper. Serve with miso or mushroom gravy as a light meal or as aside.

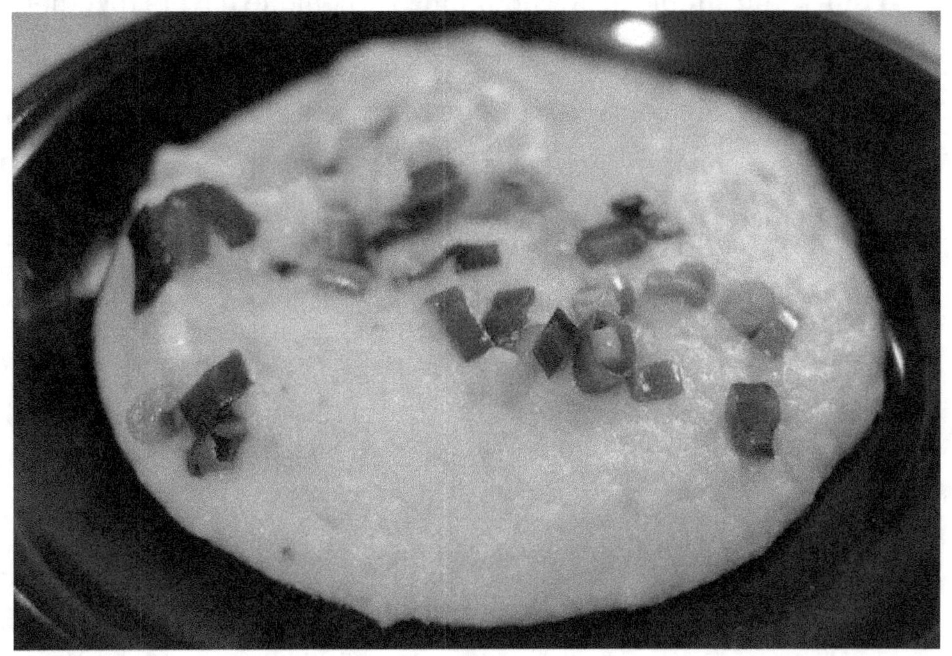

Fried Beets and Onions

A quick and simple dish, combining two unique flavors together, this dish makes a great side with a roast root vegetable or baked tofu as the main course. Just a bit of sea salt and black pepper are used to enhance these vegetables, as they produce a strong enough blend of taste on their own.

- 1 large or two small beetroot
- 1 medium onion
- 2 tablespoons of olive oil

To prepare this dish, heat a skillet on medium with olive oil. Slice the onions into fine rings and add to the pan, frying on medium or medium-low. Wash and scrub the beetroot and slice as thinly as possible, using a peeler, and add to the skillet. Fry until tender then removes and serves.

For a slight twist on this recipe, caramelize the onions and beets by adding in 1-2 teaspoons of raw sugar, coating the vegetables as much as possible. The beets and onions can serve as a unique topping for a vegetable burger or as a topping on grilled portobello mushrooms.

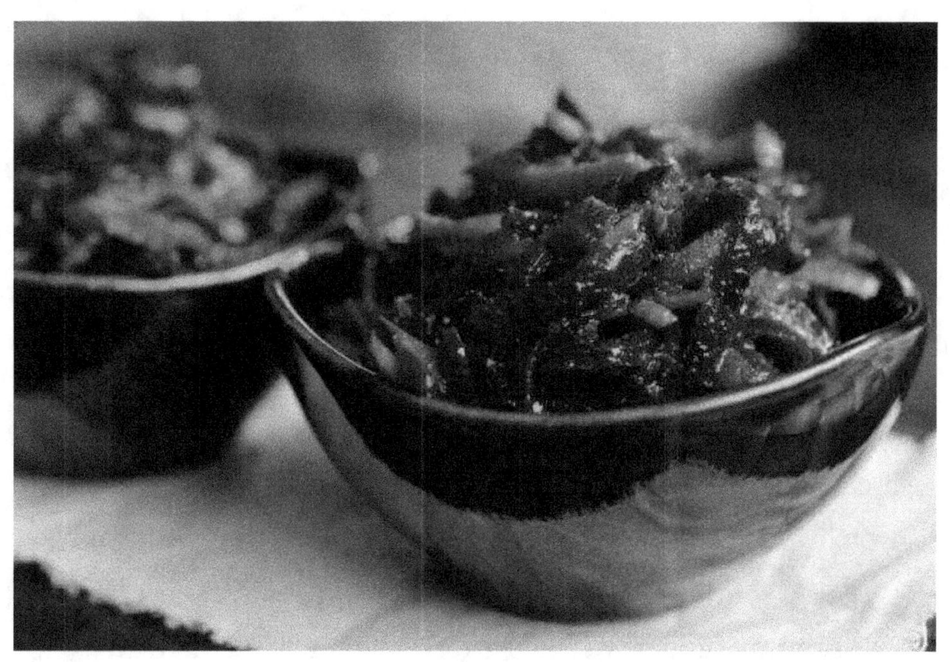

Chapter 4: Soups and Salad Recipes

Simple Broths and Soups

Sometimes a simple broth or light soup is all that's needed to satisfy your taste and offer a pleasant taste. Vegetable broth is often available in a variety of brands at the local store, and while it can be time-consuming to create your own broth, it is a worthwhile endeavor, and the health benefits are significant. Creating your own broth can be done using leftover vegetable peels, scraps, and shavings. Instead of discarding them or adding them to the compost, consider collecting them in a bag or container in the fridge or freezer, until they can be used to make a broth.

Homemade Vegetable Broth

A basic vegetable broth doesn't require a standard recipe, though there are some distinct flavors you'll want to add while creating your homemade recipe:

- Celery (leaves and/or stems)
- Carrots (peelings)

- Onions (skins, leftover slices)

- Garlic (skins, leaves pieces from cloves)

- Bay leaves

- Dried herbs

- Dark leafy green stems and leaves

- Sea salt

- Black pepper

- Seeds, peels, and stems from bell peppers and chili
  pepper

In a large cooking pot, pour 6 cups of water and combine all the vegetable peels, stems, and leftovers into the pot, then add in the salt and pepper. Bring to a boil and cook all ingredients for about ten minutes, then reduce to medium and cook for another 30 minutes before reducing to a simmer. Continue to simmer on low for several hours. A slow cooker is another way to continue simmering the broth for at least 4-5 hours. Test taste every hour or so, to determine if additional spices or herbs are needed. When the broth has reached the desired taste, remove from heat and cool for about one hour. Drain the liquid into a sturdy, resealable container and refrigerate or use for a recipe.

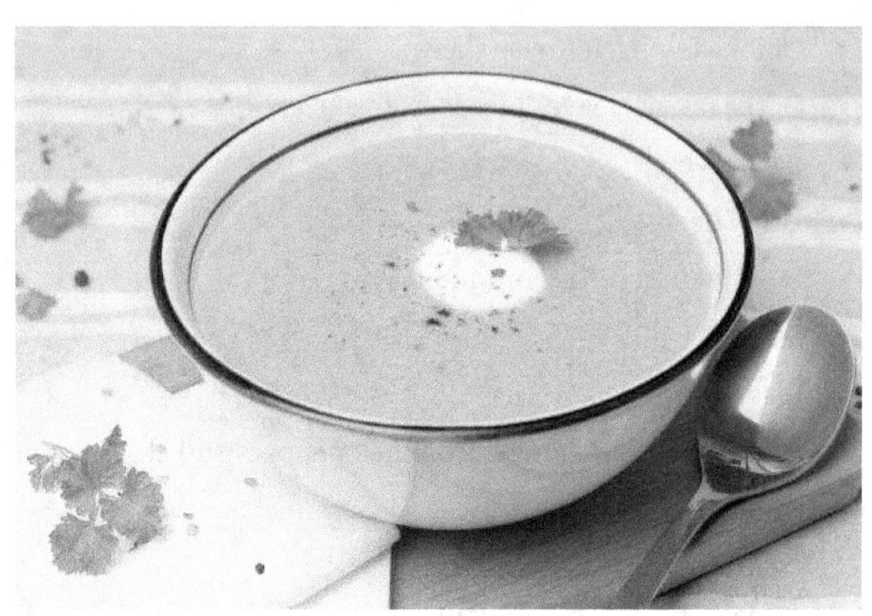

Mushroom and Miso Broth (or Soup)

This broth combines miso (a fermented soy food) with a mild broth made from sautéed mushrooms and onions. This broth is based on the above vegetable broth, with the following ingredients added:

- 2 cups of sautéed mushrooms (shitake, sliced portobello and/or button mushrooms)
- ¼ cup of miso paste

Any variety of mushrooms can be used as desired, including a blend of several types. Heat a skillet on medium heat and fry the two cups of thinly sliced mushrooms for approximately 4-5 minutes, until brown, then remove from heat. Combine the fried mushrooms with the broth and add in the ¼ cup of miso paste. Re-heat the vegetable broth, if not already on the stovetop, on medium heat, and gradually stir and combine the mushrooms and miso to blend with the broth. This will take approximately 20-25 minutes.

To serve, there are two options: keep the mushrooms in the broth and serve as a light soup, with black pepper and other seasonings. As an alternative, drain the mushrooms from the broth and prepare as a broth for another soup recipe. To create a mushroom and miso sauce or gravy, remove one cup of the broth and heat separately, mixing in two tablespoons of whole wheat flour and another tablespoon of miso paste.

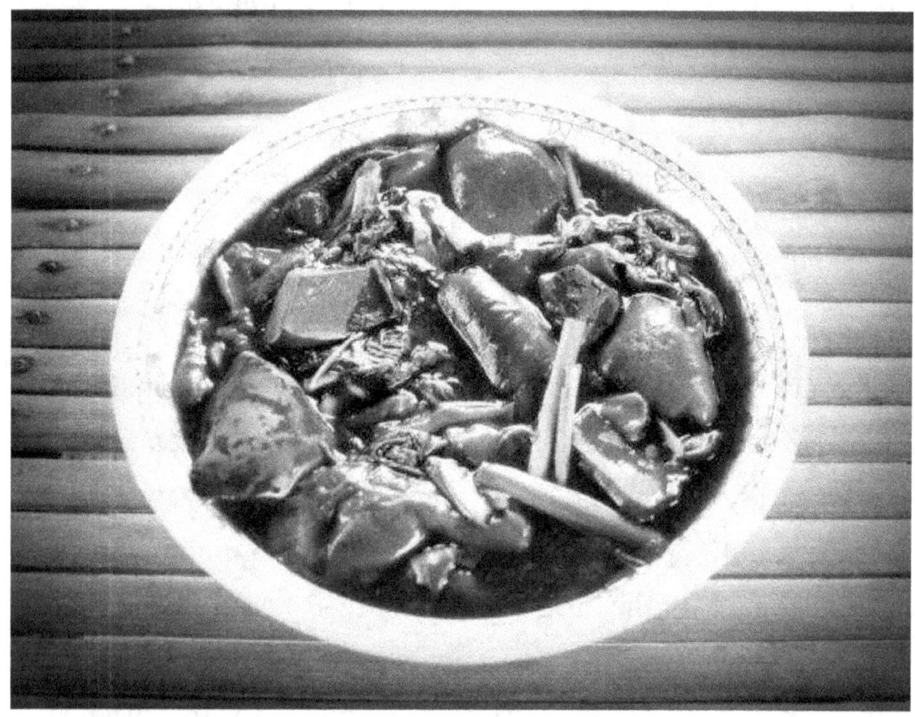

Garlic and Onion Broth

This broth is created with the vegetable broth base, by either roasting the garlic and onion in the oven or frying in a skillet and adding to the broth to cook and enhance both flavors into the soup. Roasted garlic is mild, aromatic, and provides a different taste to the soup when added. To create a thicker, more soup-like meal, blend the roasted garlic and onion with one or two cups of broth to a puree in the food processor, then return to the cooking pot and heat, stirring to thicken the remaining broth into a soup.

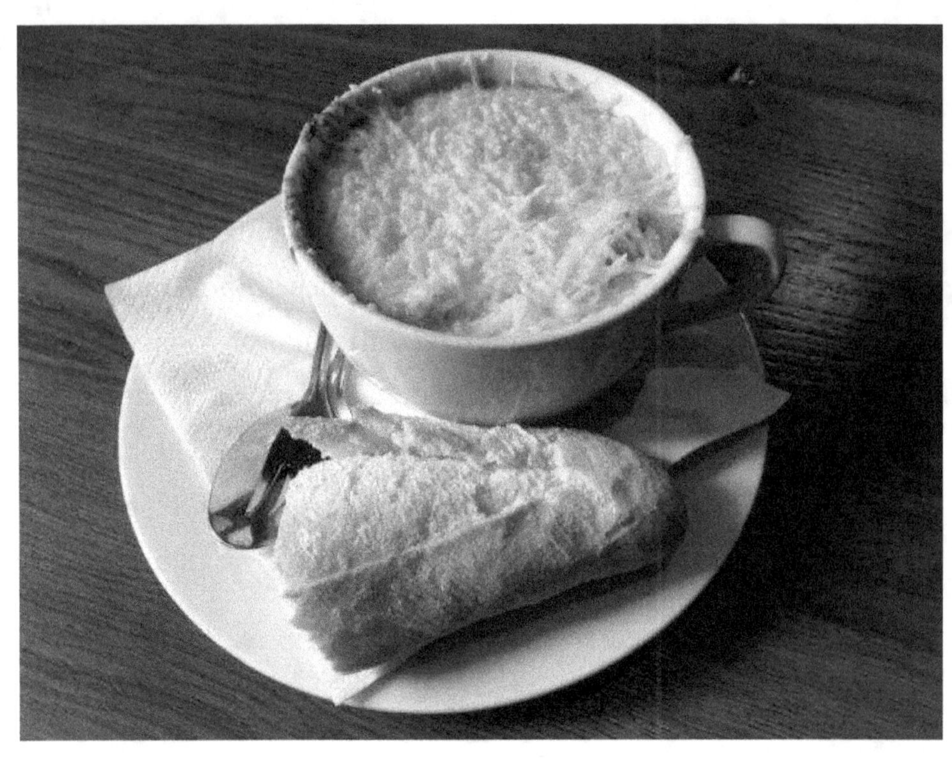

Create Your Own Soup

When creating your own soup, there are many options for ingredients to consider, in addition to the vegetables, herbs, and spices used to create the broth. The following ingredients are good ideas for customizing a soup that will fulfill not only your daily nutrients but satisfy your taste buds as well.

- Barley, quinoa, rice, and other grains are excellent for soups. Not only do they "plump" and thicken when cooked in a broth or soup, but they also soak up the flavor of the broth and the spices added. Quinoa is especially a great choice, as it contains one of the highest levels of protein of all grains, making it a good way to balance your meal.

- Tofu and tempeh, either together or separately, make a great addition to any soup. If you prefer a soft, easy texture to absorb the soup, tofu is a good option, and tempeh can be a tasty option, especially if marinated and baked beforehand, to add a stronger flavor to the texture. Tempeh is fermented, which contains B12, a nutrient rarely found in plant-based foods.

- Any variety of beans, such as kidney, pinto, black beans, as well as chickpeas and lentils make an excellent addition serving of fiber and protein to the soup. In combination with grains, beans create a full meal in the soup.

- Add some heat with sliced jalapenos, crushed dried chilis or cayenne pepper. Bell peppers, broccoli, cauliflower, okra, and other vegetables not included in the initial creation of the broth are also great to add and can take the taste options in a variety of directions.

The options for creating your own plant-based soup are plenty and will allow you to explore new food items that you might not have considered before. Soups offer a good way to "test" taste many foods we might otherwise avoid for strong flavor. Cabbage, beetroot, asparagus, and turnips are good examples of excellent soup ingredients that are not often enjoyed in their raw form, except for some salads. Potatoes and yams offer a mild yet filling ingredient to thicken and enhance soups. To create a cream soup, simply blend boiled potatoes or yams with broth and add in some plain, unsweetened soymilk.

Salads

Arugula, Cherries and Almond Salad

This salad combines the dark leafy greens of arugula with the sweetness of cherries and the texture of almonds in one dish. The nutrient value of this recipe adequate as a meal on its own. The ingredients are simple, and the dressing complements the eclectic nature of the sweet, nutty, and bitter flavors, tied together with a citrus-based vinaigrette.

- 1 bunch arugula, washed and sliced into smaller pieces
- 1 cup of slivered or sliced almonds
- ½ cup of dried cherries

For the dressing:

- ¼ cup of olive oil
- 2 tablespoons of orange or cherry marmalade
- 2 teaspoons of freshly squeezed orange or lemon

In a small bowl, combine the three ingredients to create the dressing, and set aside. In a large bowl, toss the arugula, sliced or slivered almonds, and dried cherries. Mix until all ingredients are evenly mixed. Drizzle the dressing over the salad and serve.

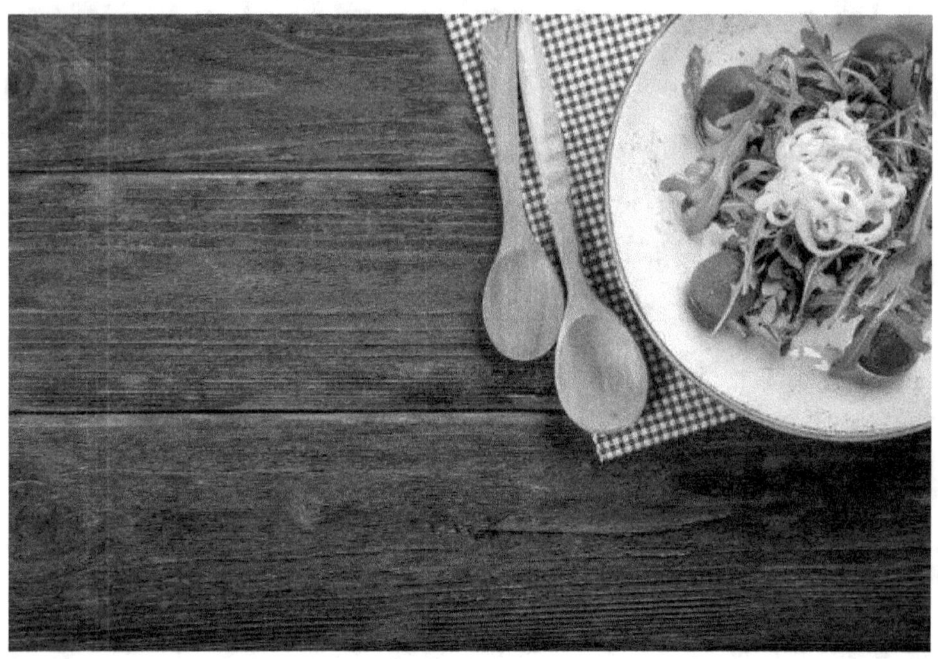

Citrus Spinach and Pecan Salad

Spinach is a great base for salad and combines well with a lot of flavors. Pecans and orange slices are added to this dish to create a tasty dish that can be enjoyed as a meal or a side dish. Mandarins or clementine oranges are also great to use for this salad, as they tend to be sweeter than regular oranges. Pecans complement the two flavors of sweet and bitter, though if unavailable, walnuts can be added as a substitute.

- 1 bunch of raw spinach, washed, rinsed, and sliced (stems removed)
- 2-3 small oranges (mandarins or clementine oranges are recommended)
- ½ cup of chopped pecans

For the dressing:

- ¼ cup of olive oil
- 2 tablespoons freshly squeezed orange juice
- 1 teaspoon maple syrup

To prepare the dressing, combine the three ingredients for the dressing and set aside. In a large bowl, toss in the spinach and pecans and mix evenly. Add in the oranges and drizzle the dressing over the salad and serve.

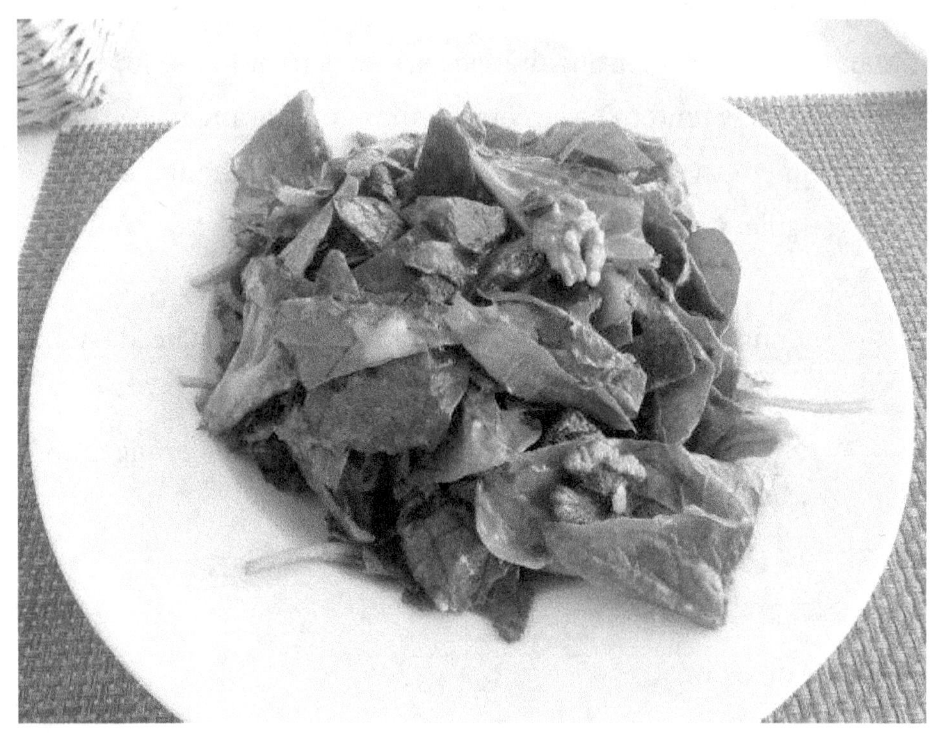

Quinoa and Parsley Salad

Parsley is often seen and used as a garnish, though it can be an excellent ingredient inside of many recipes as well. This salad combines quinoa, parsley, and a number of other ingredients to create a meal out of a salad.

- 2 cups of cooked quinoa
- 1 cup of raw, diced parsley (fresh)
- 1 teaspoon of black pepper
- 2 tablespoons dried cranberries
- ½ cup of vegan crumbled cheese
- 2 teaspoons freshly squeezed lemon juice

In a large bowl, add the cooked quinoa, parsley, and cranberries and mix well. Add in the black pepper and squeeze the lemon juice evenly over the salad. Stir in the crumbled vegan cheese and serve in bowls. If you prefer to omit the cheese or use an alternative option, crushed walnuts or pecans are a tasty topping.

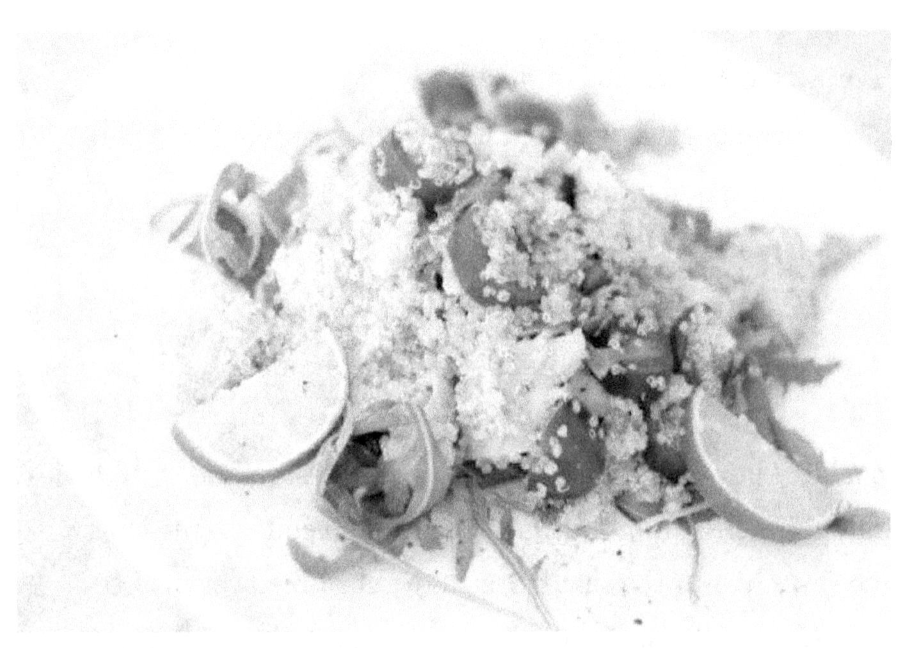

Chapter 5: Lunch Recipes

Quick Lunches on The Go

Wraps and sandwiches are often the best ways to satisfy your appetite with a portable lunch. You can create a wild range of wraps from sprouts, hummus, grilled or fried vegetables, baked tempeh or tofu, and many other ingredients.

Hummus and Sprout Wrap

Hummus is a popular chickpea-based spread that contains tahini, olive oil, and lemon. Some varieties contain chili pepper, pine nuts, beetroot, and avocado as additional flavors. This spread is popular in sandwiches and wraps, making a great substitute for meat and dairy, and an enhancement to other ingredients, such as alfalfa and mustard seed sprouts, green onions, and sliced tomatoes. This wrap is simple and easy to assemble for a quick lunch at work or on the go:

- 2 pieces of flatbread
- Hummus (any variety – plain or with a specific blend or flavor)

- 1 cup of sprouts

- 2 green onions, diced

- 1 medium tomato, sliced thinly

- Dash of black pepper

- Dash of sea salt

Arrange two wraps on plates and spread a generous layer of hummus on both. Layer with tomatoes, green onions, then sprouts. Add some black pepper and sea salt, if desired. Fold each wrap and grill, then serve.

Avocado, Basil and Tomato Wrap

Basil is a tasty herb that works well with both tomatoes and avocado. To prepare this wrap for a take-away lunch, blend some lime or lemon with the avocado after mashing it, to prevent it from going brown. If the avocado is slightly browned, it can still be used in this recipe with some added citrus to preserve the freshness. This will also add some dimension to the taste of this wrap. Fresh basil leaves are recommended, though dried work as well.

- 2 pieces of flatbread
- 1 large, ripe avocado
- 1 teaspoon of olive oil
- 2 teaspoons of lemon or lime juice
- 1 medium tomato, sliced
- 4 basil leaves (fresh, or dried)
- Dash of black pepper
- Dash of sea salt

Arrange both slices of flatbread. In a small bowl, mash the flesh of the avocado, and add in the lime or lemon juice, olive oil, and black pepper. Continue to mash and add sea salt, if desired. Spread the avocado on each bread, and layer with tomatoes, then add basil leaves and fold each wrap. Grill briefly, then serve.

Thermos Chili

If you prefer a warm meal on the commute to work or travel, this is a great option. A medium or large thermos is perfect for a fulfilling chili meal, which can be prepared the night before and warmed up in the morning. A high-quality thermos can keep food warm for a complete day, or at least until lunch.

- 2 small cans or one large can of crushed tomatoes (or puree)
- ½ cup of black beans
- ½ cup of pinto beans
- ¼ cup of kidney beans
- 2-3 tablespoons of TVP (textured vegetable protein) – optional
- 2 cloves of crushed garlic
- 1 small onion, diced
- 2 tablespoons of chili powder
- 1 teaspoon of black pepper

In a medium or large cooking pot, pour the crushed or pureed tomatoes and set aside. In a medium skillet, heat two tablespoons of olive oil and add in the onion and garlic, frying for a few minutes. Add in the chili powder and black pepper and sauté for two more minutes, then remove from heat and cool slightly, and add to the tomato sauce in the large pot. Heat on medium and stir in the three beans (ensure beans are thoroughly drained and rinsed before adding). Add in the TVP (textured vegetable protein) and stir in extra spices as desired, such as celery salt, more chili powder and/or cayenne. Cook on medium-low for 30-40 minutes, or until all ingredients are well blended and tender. Refrigerate or pour into a thermos to keep for lunch or reheat later to take away for your trip. This recipe creates approximately 3-4 servings, which makes it an ideal dish to enjoy during the week.

Additional ingredients to consider adding to this recipe include:

- Sliced, fried celery
- Shredded carrots
- Sautéed bell peppers
- Fried mushrooms
- Shredded vegan cheese
- Sliced broccoli florets

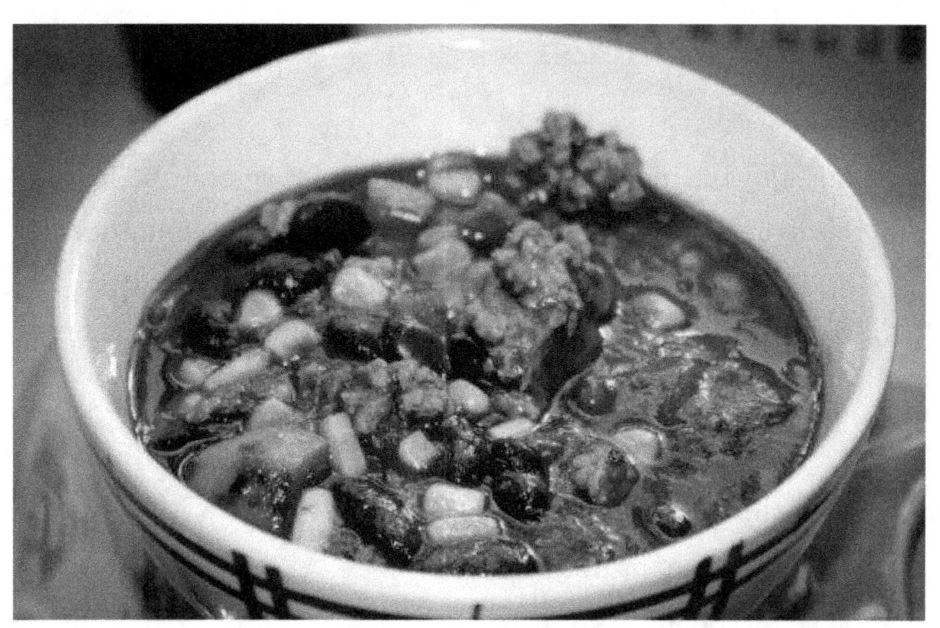

**Thermos Lentil Dal**

If you enjoy the mellow, pleasant flavors of turmeric and lentils in this dish, you'll want to take it with you on your commute to work. This is a simplified version of the lentil dal dish, which can be added to your thermos.

- 2 cups of vegetable broth
- 1 cup of lentils
- 3 tablespoons of turmeric
- 2 teaspoons of sea salt
- 2 teaspoons of olive oil
- 2 cloves of garlic, crushed
- 1 small onion, diced

In a small skillet, heat the olive oil and add in the onion and garlic. Sauté for a few minutes, then add in the turmeric. Cook for 2-3 minutes, then add to the vegetable broth and pour in the red lentils. Cook on medium for approximately 25-30 minutes, until lentils are tender. The results of the dal should resemble a soup or stew. Remove from heat and cool, then pour into a thermos. Any remaining dal can be refrigerated and used for up to one week for meals.

Home Cooked Lunch Recipes

If you take your lunch at home, there are some great vegan meal options to create, which are simple and full of flavor.

Roasted Eggplant Wrap

Roasting eggplant in your oven takes about half an hour and can be a tasty filling for a wrap or sandwich. To prepare the eggplant, slice into small disks, then wash and rinse. Lightly coat in sea salt and add to a colander. Set aside for 20 minutes, then rinse and preheat the oven to 350 degrees. Prepare a lined baking sheet greased with olive oil and place the eggplant pieces on top. Bake for approximately 25-30 minutes, until tender, then remove from the oven and set aside. To prepare the bell pepper and red onion, heat a skillet on medium with olive oil and fry for about 3-4 minutes, then set aside.

- 2 slices of flatbread
- 1 roasted eggplant (sliced, rinsed and oven-roasted)
- 1 small red onion, sliced in rings
- 1 sautéed bell pepper
- ½ cup of hummus

- 1 teaspoon of chili powder

- 1 teaspoon of sea salt

- Dash of black pepper

Arrange each flatbread and spread hummus on each slice. Top with eggplant, then fried onion rings, and bell peppers. Top with chili pepper, salt, and pepper. Fold each wrap and grill, then serve.

Vegan Grilled Cheese Deluxe

When creating a vegan grilled cheese sandwich, it's best to know which types of plant-based cheese melt better than others. Soy-based cheese tends not to melt and retains its form after the microwave or oven. Other forms of plant-based cheese, derived from vegetable oils, melt similarly to dairy cheese, and provide a great filling for this recipe. The "deluxe" part of this sandwich includes adding sliced avocado, fried onions and bell peppers with some salt and pepper.

- 1 cup of shredded or sliced vegetable-based melting cheese
- 2 slices of whole wheat bread
- 1 semi-ripe avocado, pitted, peeled, and sliced
- 1 small or medium onion, sliced in rings
- 1 bell pepper, sliced lengthwise
- Dash of sea salt
- Dash of black pepper
- 2 tablespoons of olive oil
- 1 teaspoon of vegan mayonnaise

Heat a skillet on medium and coat lightly with olive oil. Lightly sauté the onion rings and bell pepper slices for 4-5 minutes, then remove from skillet and set aside. Add the following to one slice:

- A thin spread of vegan mayonnaise
- 2 slices or the equivalent of melting vegan cheese
- Sliced avocado
- Fried onion rings
- Fried bell pepper slices

Sprinkle with salt and pepper and add the top slice. Press firmly, yet gently and add more oil to the skillet. Fry the sandwich on both sides, until toasted and cheese is melted, then slice in half and serve.

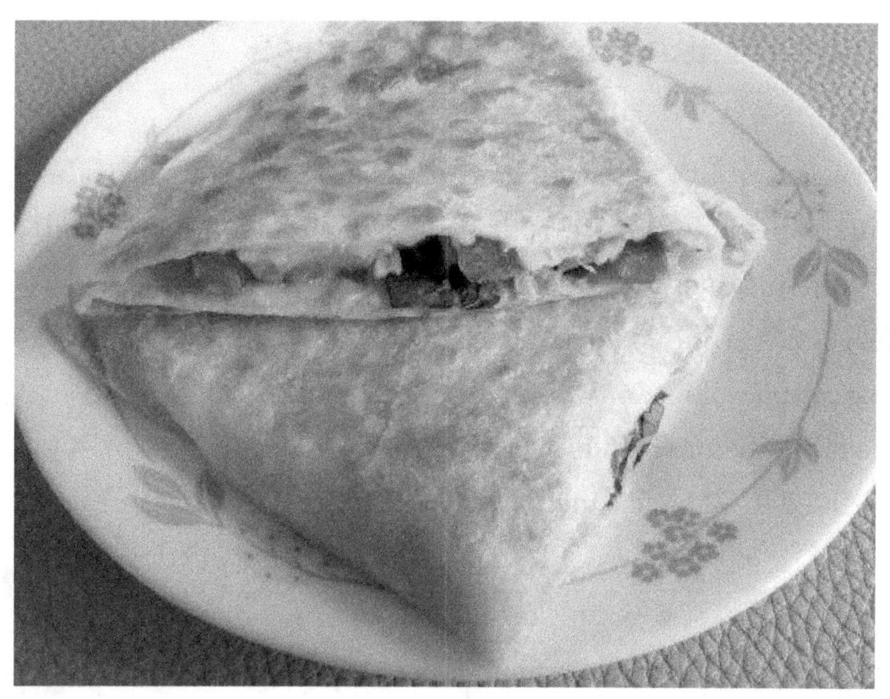

Potato Leek Soup

A warm, comfort food with lots of nutrients, this soup is made
with homemade or store-bought vegetable broth. Potatoes and
leek are the main ingredients, though other spices and
vegetables are added to enhance the flavor. The preparation of
this recipe is done in two stages: one to cook the ingredients in
the broth, before blending into a "creamy" texture, then
reheated to add a few more items.

- 4 cups of vegetable broth
- 3-4 small or medium potatoes
- 2 large leeks, sliced in 2-inch pieces (washed and rinsed)
- 1 teaspoon of black pepper
- 2 teaspoons of celery salt
- 2 carrots, sliced
- 2 teaspoons of sea salt
- 1 small onion, diced

In a large cooking pot, pour in the vegetable broth and bring to a
boil on medium-high. Wash, scrub and sliced the potatoes
(removing the skins or leaving them attached) and add to the
broth. Add in the celery salt, carrots, sea salt, onion, and black
pepper and continue to cook on medium until potatoes are
tender. Remove the pot from the stove and allow to cool. Process

in batches in a food processor or blender, until the soup, is smooth and creamy. Return to the large pot and reheat, then stir in the leaks. Serve with a dollop of vegan sour cream and meatless bacon bits.

If leek is not in season and you'd like to make this soup, try substituting green onion or fresh dill instead. Creamy potato soup can be modified for many other ingredients, including chopped spinach, slices of smoked tofu or tempeh and parsley.

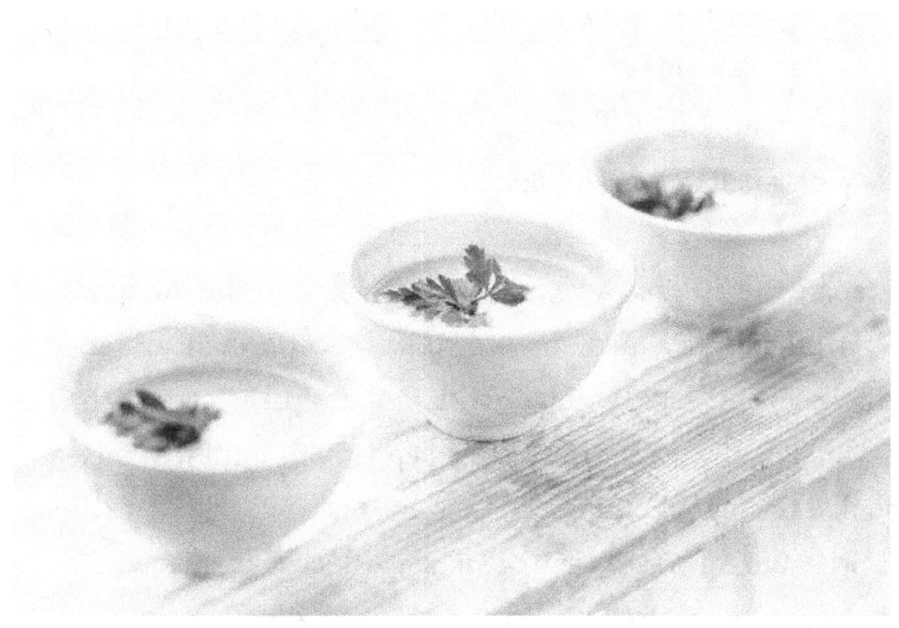

Turnip Patties

A simple and easy side recipe or a light meal, turnips are a root
vegetable that can be baked and fried like a potato. Their texture
is a bit tougher than potatoes or yams, though they soften and
mellow in the oven during a roast or can be shredded or sliced
for the frying pan. For this recipe, turnips (also called rutabaga)
are shredded using a large grater and transferred into a bowl
and formed with a few ingredients to create patties.

- 2 medium or 3 small turnips
- 2 tablespoons of soymilk
- 2 tablespoons of whole wheat flour
- 2 teaspoons of sea salt
- 1 teaspoon of black pepper
- 1 small onion, shredded

Prepare the turnips by removing the stems and shredding with a
large grater into a medium-sized bowl. Using a small grater,
shred the onion and combine with the turnip, then stir in the
soymilk, flour, sea salt, and black pepper. Stir until well mixed,
so that the ingredients stick together. If needed, add more milk
or wheat to thin or thicken the mix. Heat a skillet on medium
with olive oil and form one patty (3-4 inches in diameter) and
fry on each side carefully, to avoid breaking the patty apart. Fry

on each side for 3-4 minutes until golden brown, then serve with vegan sour cream and/or salsa or guacamole. Patties can be served on their own with a dash of chili pepper or as a side with a meal.

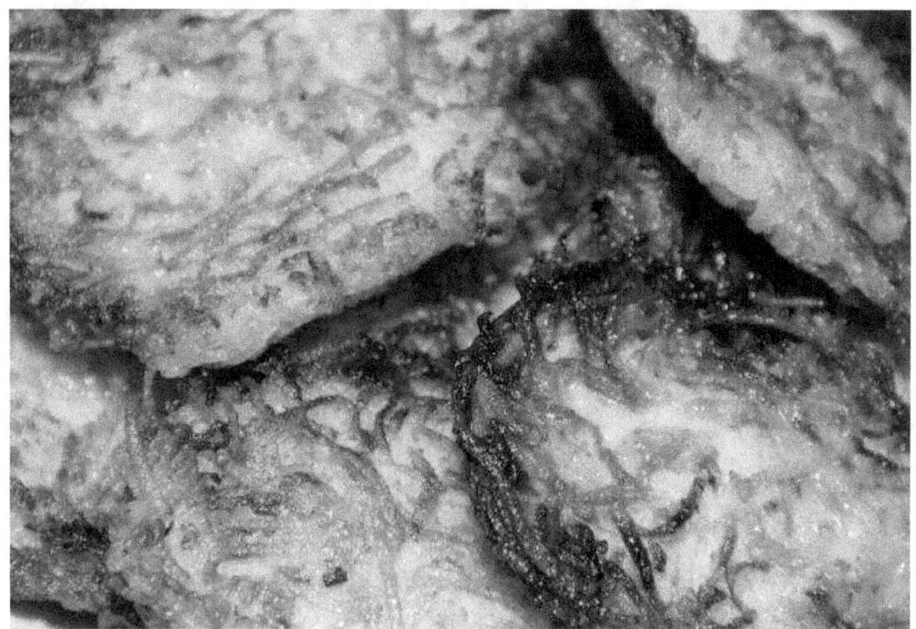

Chapter 6: Dinner Recipes

Plant-Based Meals for Dinner

Vegetarian Shepherd's Pie

This recipe is prepared in a large casserole dish and includes a variety of root vegetables, along with a soy-based "meat" alternative. If a soy-based ground "meat" is not desired or available, lentils are added to boost the protein content of this meal. Adding both may also be considered, and this will add more texture to the layers. The top layer of shepherd's pie is traditionally covered in mashed potatoes, which is done similarly here as well, only with a combination of both regular and sweet potatoes.

- 1 cup of uncooked brown lentils
- 1 small package of vegan ground "meat"
- 2 large potatoes
- 2 large sweet potatoes
- 2 cloves of garlic
- 1 teaspoon of fresh dill (or dried)

- 1 teaspoon of black pepper
- 1 teaspoon of chili powder
- Dash of sea salt
- 2 large carrots, sliced in small pieces
- 2 stalks of celery, sliced in small pieces
- 1 small onion, diced
- ½ cup of corn
- ½ cup of green peas
- 2 tablespoons of whole wheat flour
- 1 tablespoon of water
- 3-4 tablespoons of soymilk (unflavored, unsweetened)

Begin this recipe by preheating the oven to 350 degrees and grease a medium to a large baking loaf pan, then set aside. On the stovetop, heat a large skillet with olive oil, and toss in the onion, garlic, and black pepper. Sauté for a few minutes, then add in the vegan ground "meat" and continue to cook. Add in the sea salt and chili powder and continue to cook on medium until brown. If the vegan meat is to be omitted, cook the one cup of lentils in two cups of boiling water, adding sea salt, then drain and add to the skillet in place of (or in addition to) the ground "meat". When this step is done, add in the corn, peas, carrots, and celery and continue to fry on medium under vegetables are tender, then gently stir in two tablespoons of whole wheat flour, followed by one tablespoon of water. Prepare a large casserole dish and grease it lightly. Scoop the vegetable and lentil mix from the skillet and layer the bottom of the dish evenly. To prepare the top layer, mash the yams in a large bowl, add in 3-4 tablespoons of soymilk and 3 tablespoons of vegan butter and mash together until smooth. Scoop and gently layer over the vegetable mix on the bottom of the dish. Ensure this layer is evenly spread, then top with black pepper, sea salt, and paprika. Bake for 30-35 minutes until the top is slightly golden. Remove and slice to serve.

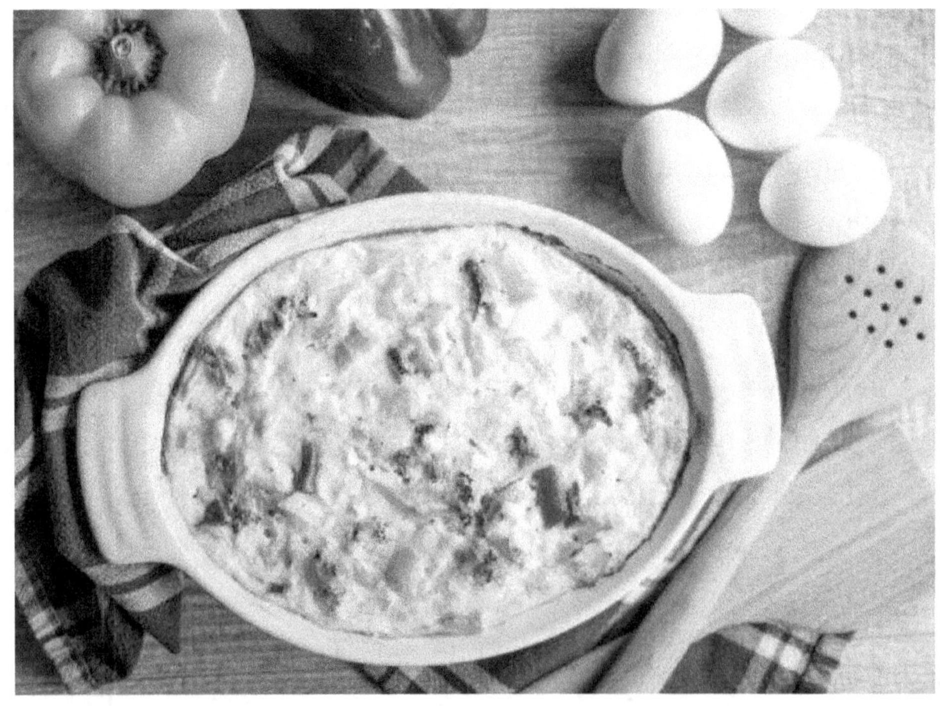

Tempeh in Tomato Sauce with Spaghetti

Tempeh is a textured, fermented soy that makes an excellent meat replacement in many meals. In this recipe, tempeh is marinated in tomato sauce and spices overnight, or for a minimum of two hours, to enhance the flavor, prior to frying and stewing with crushed tomatoes, which creates a stronger taste. The remainder of this recipe is easy and involves stewing the tomato sauce with spices and the tempeh.

- 1 block of tempeh (plain, unflavored)
- 1 large can of pureed tomatoes
- 2 tablespoons of oregano
- 1 tablespoon of thyme
- 1 teaspoon of chili powder
- 1 teaspoon of black pepper
- 2 cloves of garlic, crushed
- 1 small onion, diced
- ½ package of spaghetti noodles

In a small skillet, heat the olive oil and combine the onion and garlic. Sauté for a few minutes and add in the marinated tempeh and ½ cup of the tomato sauce. Reduce heat and simmer for 8-10 minutes, then remove. In a large cooking pot, pour the contents of the skillet with the remainder of the tomato sauce.

Heat and stir slowly on medium, though avoid bringing to a boil. Stir in the oregano, thyme, chili powder, black pepper, and salt. Blend and cook for another 15-20 minutes. Prepare the spaghetti by boiling 3-4 cups of water in a second cooking pot and add sea salt. Add the spaghetti and cook until tender, then drain and rinse. Serve the tempeh and tomato sauce over the noodles and top with vegan parmesan or garnish with fresh parsley.

Roasted Root Vegetables in a Miso Sauce

Root vegetables can create a hearty, filling meal for dinner, and as leftovers, they can easily be reheated and enjoyed at any time. Carrots, parsnips, rutabaga, yams, and potatoes are all excellent sources of fiber, and vitamin C. Radishes and beets are also good options, and although they both have strong, pungent flavors, they mellow significantly when roasted in the oven, and mix well with other vegetables. To add a good portion of protein to this meal, a simple miso sauce is made with vegetable broth and a dash of soy sauce.

- 2 large carrots, peeled and sliced lengthwise
- 2-3 parsnips, peeled and sliced lengthwise
- 1 cup of radishes, washed, scrubbed and stems removed
- 2 medium yams, sliced into large chunks (quarters)
- 1 small rutabaga, sliced into quarters
- 1 beet, sliced into one-inch-thick slices
- Fresh parsley to garnish

Miso Sauce:

- 1 cup of vegetable broth
- 1 teaspoon of soy sauce
- 1 tablespoon of miso paste

To prepare the vegetables, preheat the oven to 350 degrees and grease a deep baking dish lightly with olive oil. Add all the vegetables to the pan and set aside. In a saucepan, add the vegetable broth and bring to a boil, then stir in the miso paste and soy sauce, whisking while reducing heat to low to simmer. Pour half of the miso sauce over the vegetables, then place in the oven and bake for 30-40 minutes, or until all vegetables are tender, then pour the remaining sauce on the vegetables, and cook for another 15-20 minutes, then remove and cool slightly before serving with parsley.

Green Pea Pie

While some may consider this dish a dessert (if sweetened), or a treat, it is hearty enough for a meal as well. Green peas are not only sweet and tasty, but they are also high in protein and fiber and are easy to work within this recipe. This recipe can be prepared with pre-made vegan pie shells, or with homemade pie, shells are following:

- 1 cup of almond flour
- 2 -3 tablespoons of vegan butter

In a small bowl, mash the flour and butter together, until crumbly. Press into a pie tin to evenly coat the entire pan, including the sides. Bake in the oven for 10-12 minutes at 350, then remove, cool, and set aside. The following ingredients are combined to create the green pea filling:

- 2 cups of fresh green peas
- 1 teaspoon of raw sugar
- 3-4 tablespoons of vegan butter
- 2 tablespoons of parsley
- 2 tablespoons of dill
- ½ teaspoons of black pepper
- Dash of sea salt

- 1 tablespoon of vegetable broth

In a large cooking pot, shell green peas and cook in water. Bring to a boil, add some vegan butter, salt, raw sugar and reduce heat. Continue to cook on medium. Stir in dill, parsley and vegetable broth and cook until done, but still bright green in color. Remove from the stove and cool. If desired, mash the peas, or leave them whole. Scoop the peas into the pie shell. Bake in the oven for 15-20 minutes, then cool, slice and serve.

Chapter 7: Dessert Recipes

Puddings and Ice Cream

Easy to make and enjoy, puddings and ice cream don't require too much preparation, and can be modified to include all plant-based ingredients and nutrients. During your shopping trips, you may notice a variety of soft or silken tofu, with some varieties or brands offering flavored tofu pudding desserts. These can also be made at home with the right amount of ingredients, including a natural sweetener and flavors or your choice. Other pudding bases include milk and chia seeds. Chia seeds are high in protein, antioxidants, calcium, fiber and make it easy to get those daily nutrient requirements into your diet. When chia seeds are soaked in milk, they soften, become gel-like, and create a pudding texture that can be added to fruits, cocoa, and a variety of nuts. Many people who follow a low carb, ketogenic or paleo diet love chia seeds because they are low in carbs and high in nutrients.

Mango Tofu Pudding

The next time you venture past the tofu and meat alternative section of your grocery store, consider buying a package of silken tofu. It's a great based for dessert, and you find it easy to work with, as it blends well in a food processor. When choosing a brand of silken tofu, choose unsweetened, unflavored, and if available, organic.

- 1 large or 2 small ripe mangoes
- 2 teaspoons of maple syrup
- 1 package of silken tofu, drained

Combine all three ingredients into a blender or food processor and pulse until smooth. If the pudding is too thick, add one or two tablespoons of coconut or almond milk to thin. Serve in dessert bowls. This treat will last up to three days in the refrigerator.

Coconut Tofu and Pistachio Pudding

This recipe can be prepared with either a coconut flavored silken tofu (or package of coconut tofu pudding), or the plain, unflavored soft tofu. Coconut milk or cream, and shredded coconut are added with crushed pistachios to create a textured, tasty snack.

- 1 package of silken tofu, drained (plain or coconut flavor)
- ½ cup of coconut milk or cream
- ¼ cup of shredded coconut (unsweetened)
- ¼ cup of crushed pistachios
- 2 teaspoons of raw sugar or coconut sugar

Combine the tofu and milk together in a food processor and blend until smooth. Add in the shredded coconut, sweetener, and pistachios and continue to pulse. Serve with additional shredded coconut and/or crushed pistachios on top. If pistachios are not available, substitute with peanuts or walnuts.

Basic Chia Seed Pudding

This pudding is created with two main ingredients: non-dairy milk and chia seeds. A basic chia seed pudding consists of three main ingredients:

- ½ cup of chia seeds
- 3 tablespoons of maple syrup or low carb sweetener
- 1 ½ cups of almond or coconut milk

Combine all three ingredients together in a container and refrigerate for at least two hours. Chia seeds will gently soften and expand in milk, and become jelly-like, creating an ideal pudding texture. The sweetener enhances the blend of chia seeds and milk, which can be enjoyed on its own as a simple, no-frills dessert, or a base for toppings and other ingredients. Add a dash of vanilla extract to the chia pudding for flavor.

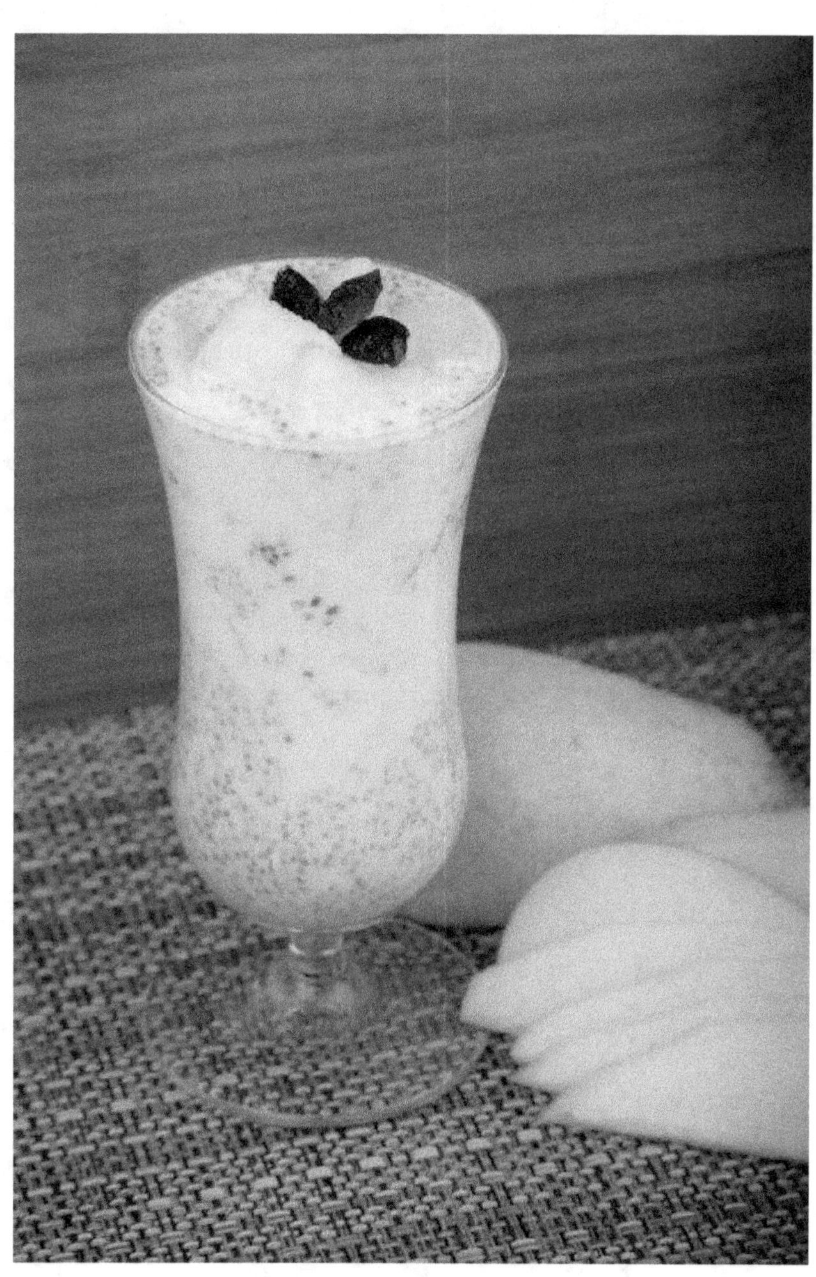

Raspberry Chia Seed Pudding

To create raspberry chia seed pudding, add one cup of frozen or fresh raspberries to the milk and blend in a food processor, prior to mixing with other ingredients. As an alternative, raspberries can be added after a basic chia seed pudding is prepared, as a topping, or folded into the pudding.

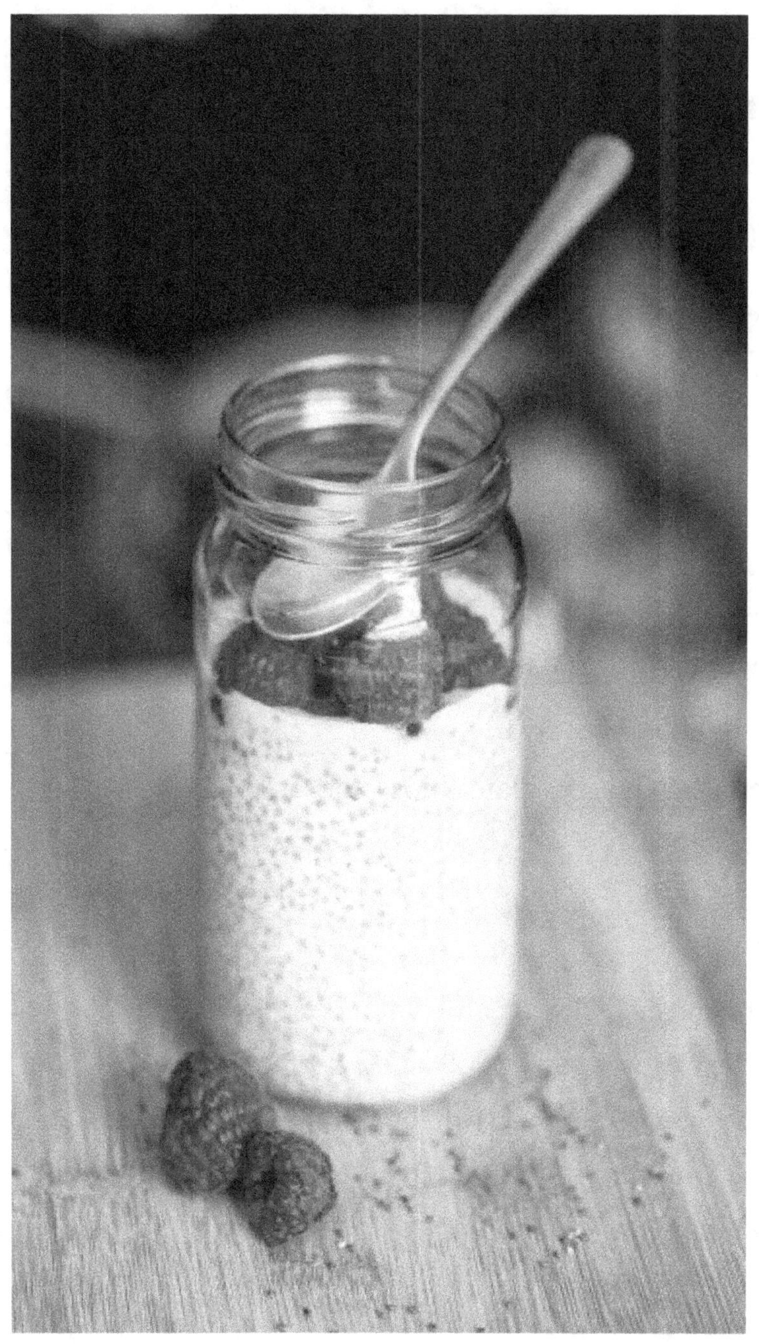

Chia Seed Pudding with Banana and Chocolate

Another fun way to experiment with chia seed pudding is by adding some raw cocoa and banana, for a decadent treat. To prepare, add half a banana to one cup of milk and blend for 30 seconds or until smooth. Add another ½ cup of almond milk and combine with chia seeds and sweetener. To create this recipe, combine the following ingredients:

- 1 cup of almond milk combined with a mashed banana
- ½ cup of almond milk
- ½ cup of chia seeds
- ¼ cup of mini chocolate chips (non-dairy, dark chocolate)
- 2 teaspoons of maple syrup or low carb sweetener

Combine the mashed banana and almond milk with the chia seeds and the extra ½ cup of milk and sweetener. Mix well, and refrigerate for a minimum of two hours, then fold the chocolate chips into the pudding before serving. Top with cocoa powder or chocolate chips.

Ice Cream

Creating an ice cream has never been easier. The following recipes include a few ingredients each and can be blended and frozen easily for any occasion.

Banana-Strawberry Ice Cream

This ice cream recipe uses bananas as a base, which can be frozen before or after. To create this recipe from frozen bananas, slice two ripe bananas into 2-inch chunks and freeze for at least two hours. Remove from the freezer and add to the blender with the following ingredients:

- 2 frozen, chopped bananas
- 1 cup of sliced strawberries (fresh or frozen)
- ½ cup of coconut milk
- 1 teaspoon of natural sweetener

Add all the ingredients to a blender and pulse for 45 seconds until smooth and thick. Scoop into a bowl and serve.

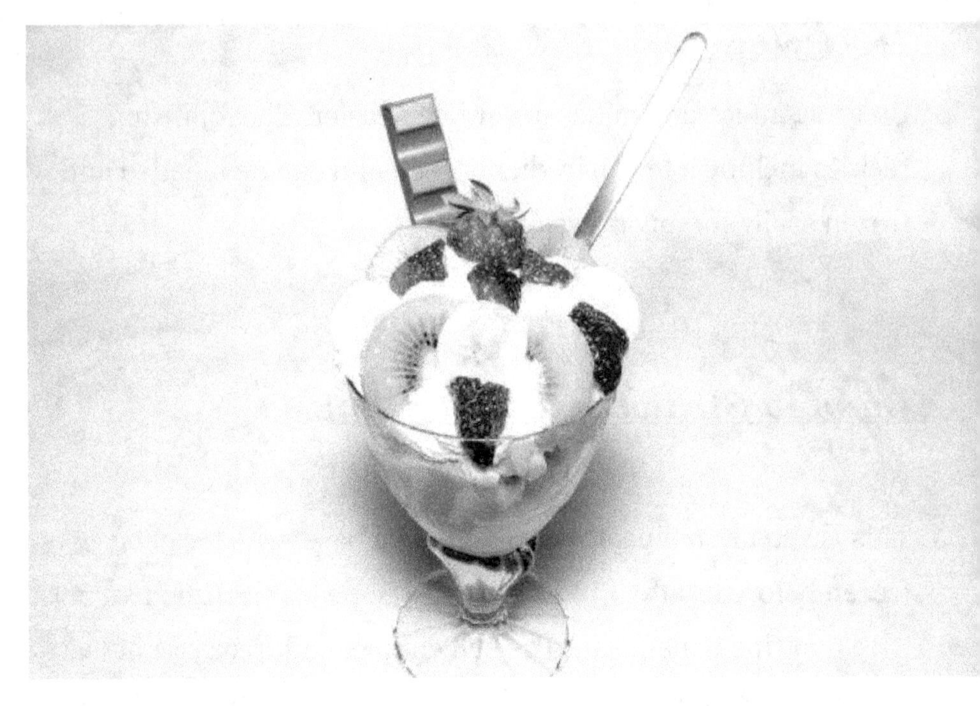

Cocoa Coconut Ice Cream

A rich tasting treat, coconut milk creates a creamier taste by combining cocoa powder, shredded coconut, and coconut oil to enhance not only the flavor but also the nutrient value.

- 2 cups of coconut milk
- ½ cup of shredded coconut
- 1 tablespoon of coconut oil
- 2 teaspoons of coconut sugar (or raw sugar)
- 2 tablespoons of cocoa powder

In a small bowl, combine the coconut milk with shredded coconut, oil, and sugar, and whisk thoroughly until well mixed. Stir in the cocoa powder and mix to combine evenly. If needed, add in more cocoa powder and blend. Pour the ingredients into a small resealable container and place it in the freezer for at least two hours. Remove to serve. If the ice cream is difficult to scoop initially after freezing, allow it to sit for 8-10 minutes before serving. Add a topping of toasted coconut flakes.

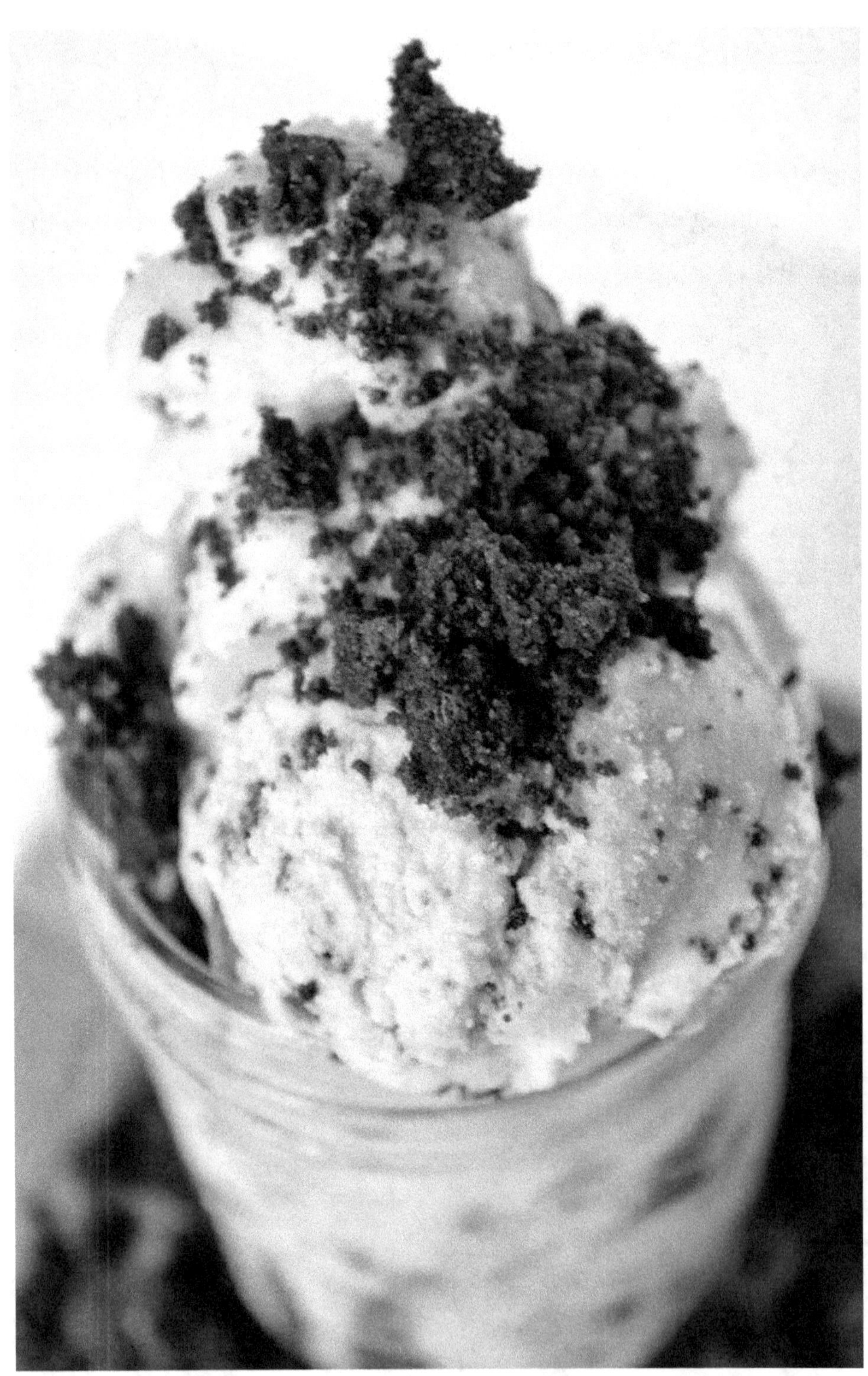

Banana, Cherry, and Mango Ice Cream

This fruit medley creates a sorbet-like ice cream that can be enjoyed in the summer or as a light dessert after a meal. To create this dessert, slice the banana into chunks and refrigerate for two hours, then remove and blend with the following ingredients.

- 2 frozen bananas, sliced into chunks
- 1 cup of pitted cherries
- 1 small or medium mango, peeled, cored, and sliced

For best results, freeze just the banana, or one of the other fruits, and combine in a food processor to create this dessert. If the fruits are too solid to blend well, add in one cup of naturally squeezed fruit juice or soy, almond or coconut milk.

Cakes and Brownies

Creating a plant-based cake or brownie is simple and doesn't require any special ingredients, as most items can already be found in your pantry. The most common differences between plant-based desserts and their regular versions are milk (usually nut-based milk, soy, or coconut milk), and avoiding any gelatin, honey or other ingredients that are animal byproducts or contain them. If you are new to vegan baking, try a few simple recipes to become familiar with the variety and type of items you'll need. Brownies are a good example of a simple or easy baked treat to start.

Vegan Brownies

Dark chocolate is the main feature of this delicious brownie recipe. These brownies are not too dry or too sweet. They are moist and contain a satisfying chocolate fix with each bite.

- 1 cup of flour
- 2 tablespoons of maple syrup or raw sugar
- ¼ cup of cocoa powder
- ½ cup of dark chocolate

- 3 tablespoons of olive oil
- 1 cup of almond milk
- ½ cup of chocolate chips (vegan)
- 1 teaspoon of vanilla extract

Prepare the oven by preheating to 350 degrees and grease a baking dish. In a medium saucepan, melt the chocolate in the cup of almond milk with vanilla. In a large bowl, mix the dry ingredients and set aside. When the chocolate is fully melted into the milk, pour into the bowl of cocoa powder, flour, and sweetener, and pour in the oil. Mix thoroughly and pour into the prepared baking dish. Gently fold in chocolate chips. Bake for 25-30 minutes or until done. Test with a fork or toothpick by pressing into the brownie. If it's clear when removed, the dish is ready to serve. Cool slightly after removing from the oven, slice and serve.

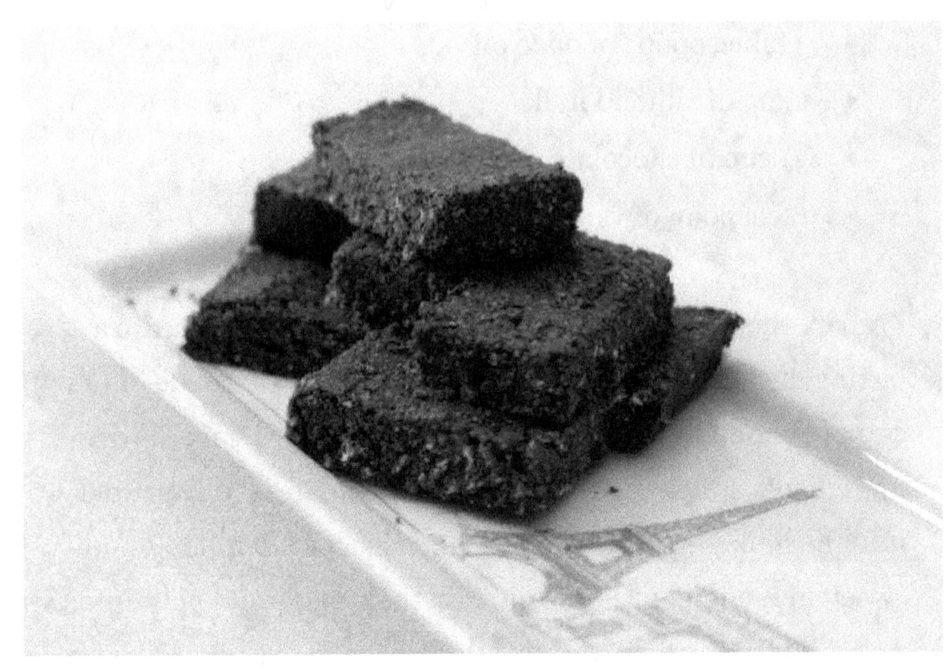

Vegan Sponge Cake

A light and tasty treat, sponge cake is a simple way to end a meal as a plain dessert or with a fruit topping. Traditionally, sponge cake includes many dairy ingredients, which are replaced with vegan-friendly versions of each, including butter, milk, and yogurt.

- ½ cup of vegan butter
- 1 cup of raw sugar
- 2 teaspoons of vanilla extract
- ½ cup of soymilk
- ½ cup of soy or another non-dairy yogurt
- 3 cups of flour
- 1 teaspoon of baking soda
- 1 teaspoon of baking powder

In a large bowl, add the dry ingredients together and blend well. In a small bowl, combine the yogurt, milk, vanilla extract, and vegan butter. When both sets of ingredients are mixed well, combine in one bowl into a batter. Preheat the oven to 325 degrees and prepare a cake tin with parchment paper and a light coating of olive oil. Pour the batter into the pan and bake for 35-40 minutes or until done. The texture should be slightly brown and spongy. Serve plain, or topped with fruit, coconut cream or other toppings such as chocolate sauce and/or maple syrup.

Create two layers of sponge cake and add a filling in the middle, such as orange marmalade, black currant jam, strawberry sauce or another fruit or nut butter filling. There are many variations to try with this cake recipe, along with unlimited options for fillings and toppings.

Almond Raspberry Orange Cake

This is a tasty fruit-filled cake with an almond twist. A small portion of hemp or flax seeds is added to add a dose of protein and healthy fats to this dessert.

- 1 ½ cups of flour (gluten-free flour can be used for this recipe)
- 2 teaspoons of baking powder
- 1 cup of sliced almonds
- ¾ cups of coconut or almond milk
- 1 teaspoon of baking soda
- ¼ cup of freshly squeezed orange juice
- ½ cup of raw sugar
- 2 teaspoons of apple cider vinegar
- ½ teaspoon of lemon or orange zest
- 1 teaspoon of vanilla extract
- 1 teaspoon of ground flax or hemp seeds
- ½ cup of fresh raspberries

Prepare a cake tin with a light coating of oil, then set aside and heat the oven to 350 degrees. In a medium bowl, combine the flour, sliced almonds, baking powder, and baking soda. Combine the following items in a second bowl: orange juice, oil, sugar, vanilla extract, lemon or orange zest, flax or hemp seeds, and vinegar. Mix both sets of ingredients carefully, folding gently and not mixing too vigorously. Pour into the cake tin and place the raspberries over the top. Add a handful of sliced almonds in between the berries. Bake in the oven for 45-50 minutes, then remove to cool. Slice and serve each slice with coconut whipped cream.

Chapter 8: Drink Recipes

Cold Beverages

There are plenty of tasty, healthy plant-based options for cold, refreshing beverages to replace the soda and high sugar content of store-bought fruit juice. Investing in an electric juicer is a great investment that can prepare a wide range of vegetable and fruit juice drinks or a combination of both. Many juicers are available in hardware or appliance stores, from a simple press to more elaborate versions of this device. Some of the recipes in this chapter can also be made without the use of a juicer.

Pomegranate Lemonade

A refreshing drink in the summer, this variation on lemonade includes adding pomegranate juice in addition to freshly squeezed lemons. To create this juice, a manual press is needed to extract the lemon juice and sweetened with maple syrup or another natural sweetener. Pomegranates tend to release their juice easily, and there is the option to add the seeds into the juice or save them for another recipe (they make excellent salad toppings)

- 3-4 freshly squeezed lemons
- 1 large pomegranate
- 1-2 teaspoons of maple syrup or raw sugar

Press the lemons, one at a time, and squeeze the juice into a cup. Repeat with the pomegranate, adding in the seeds with the juice. If the seeds are not desired, strain to remove, and mix the lemon and pomegranate juices together, stirring in the maple syrup or desired sweetener.

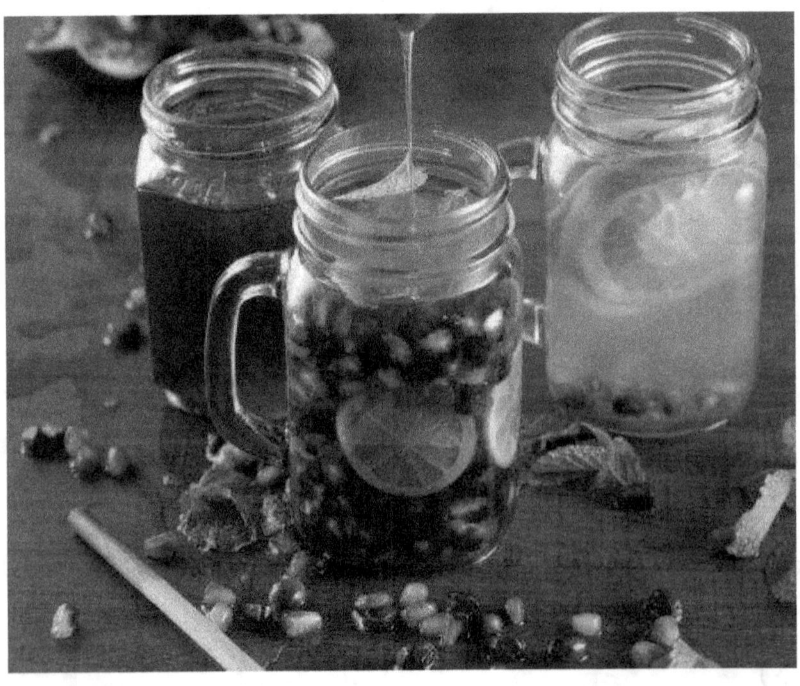

Mango Carrot Juice

If you have an electric juicer, this is a juice combination you'll want to try. The distinct flavors and natural sweetness of both mangoes and carrots are blended to create a tasty and satisfying drink to enjoy with any meal of the day. Choose a fresh, ripe mango with soft flesh inside for best results.

- 1 large or 2 medium mangos, peeled, pitted, and sliced
- 3 large carrots, stems removed

Place the slices of mango in an electric juicer, and press them into the feeder, followed by the carrots. Serve immediately. For added sweetness, squeeze one or two oranges and add to the mango carrot juice.

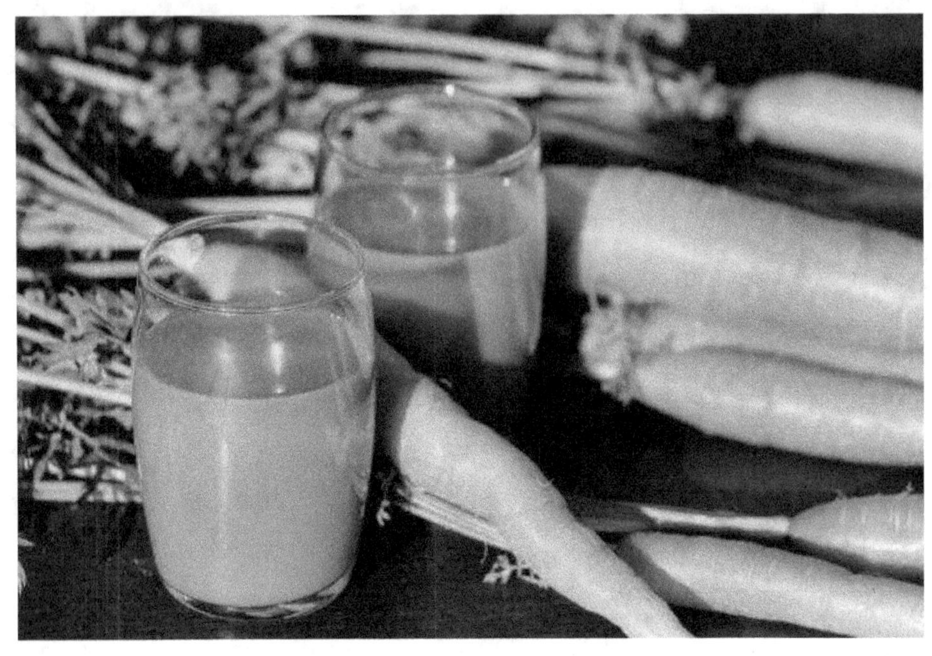

<u>Green Veggie Drink</u>

This is a great way to put your juicer to work and combine a few dark leafy greens into your diet. If you're not in the habit of enjoying kale, spinach, arugula, or parsley, you may want to add a handful of these dark greens into the juicer, along with some apple, carrot, and celery to balance the sweet and bitter flavors combined. This recipe combines all four leafy greens, though if only one or two are available, increase the portion of the combined vegetables to equal approximately three cups or slightly more.

- 1 cup of sliced kale
- 1 cup of uncooked spinach
- ½ cup of parsley
- ½ or arugula
- 2 carrots
- 2 apples
- ½ inch of ginger (optional)

In a juicer, start by feeding through the kale, spinach, parsley, and arugula and press down a carrot to follow, then ginger (optional, if using) and the apples. Add more apple or carrot if desired, to create more sweetness or to balance the flavors. Orange juice can also be added.

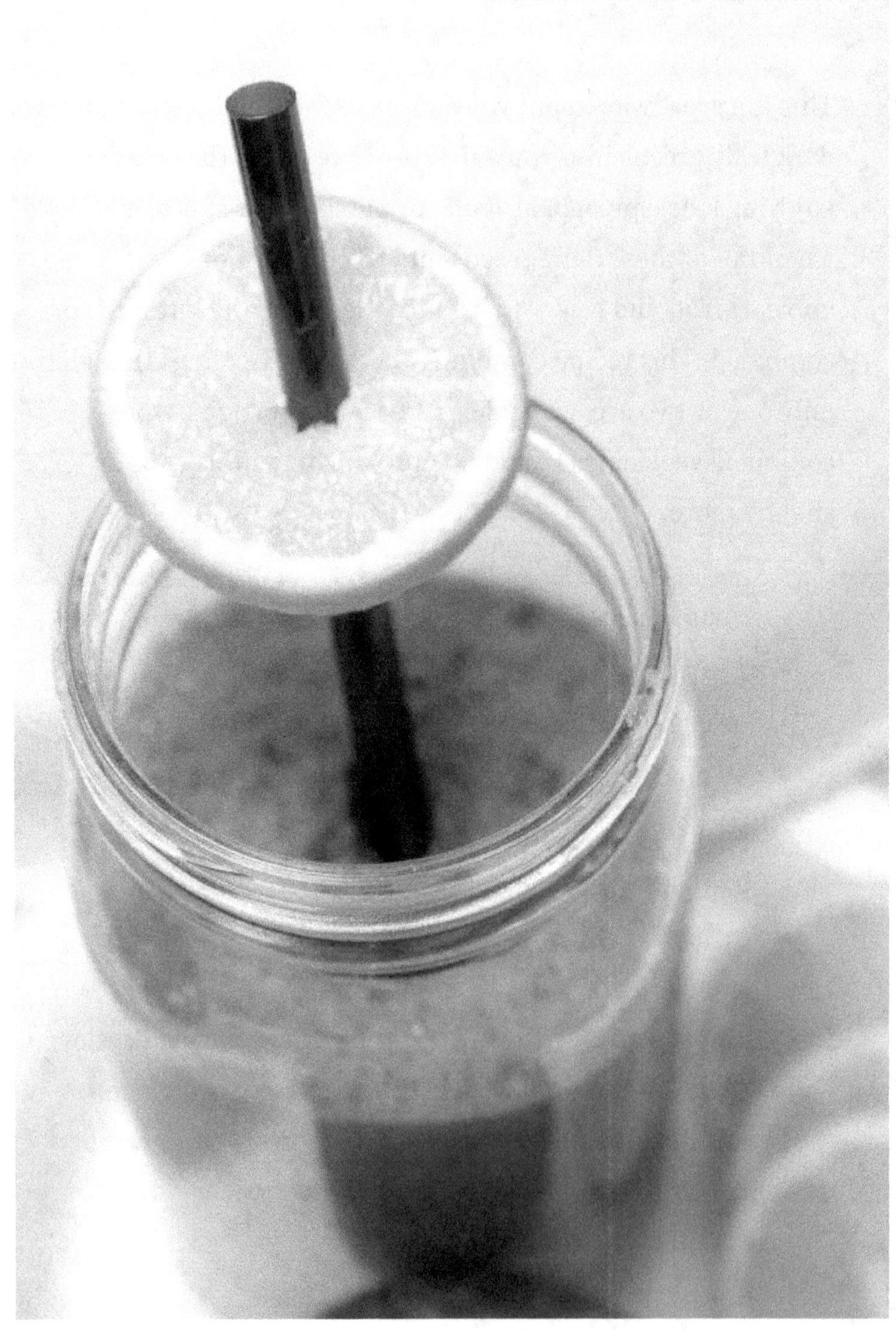

Turmeric Lemon and Orange Juice

Turmeric is a great tasting root to add into juice, and like ginger, it's a good way to naturally boost your health and immune system. One of the featured advantages of turmeric is its ability to fight and prevent inflammation, caused by chronic conditions.

- 1 inch of turmeric root
- 2 lemons
- 2-3 oranges
- 1-2 apples

To prepare this drink, add the turmeric root into the juicer, followed by the apple, then manually press the oranges and lemons, mixing them together in a bowl. Combine the turmeric-apple blend with the orange and lemon juice, then stir and enjoy. If desired, add a teaspoon of maple syrup.

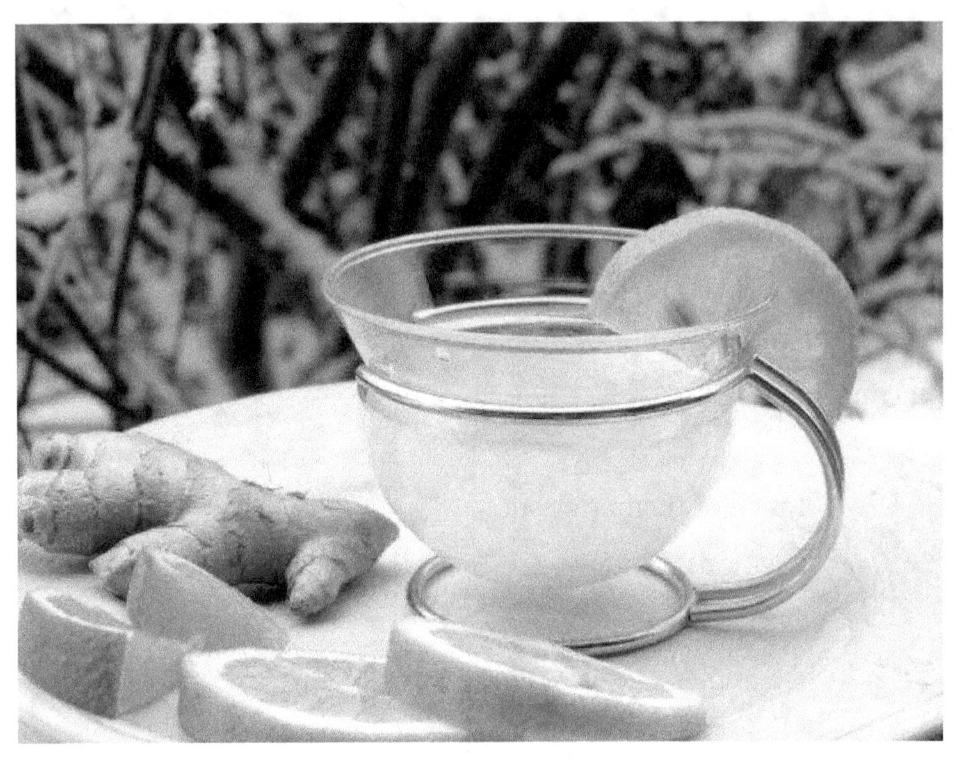

Hot Beverages

Freshly brewed coffee and steeped tea are usual favorites for hot drinks, though there are a few tasty options to consider in addition to the regular warm beverages, which infuse some spice and flavored teas for an alternative. Chai and turmeric spice, as well as green tea and herbal blends.

Warm Almond Milk with Turmeric

A strong anti-inflammatory with a high number of antioxidants, turmeric is mellow tasting root, also available as a powder for a wide variety of recipes. In this drink, turmeric is whisked with a natural sweetener.

- 2 cups of almond milk
- 2 tablespoons of turmeric
- 2 tablespoons of low carb sweetener or maple syrup
- Dash of black pepper

In a medium saucepan combine the almond milk with turmeric, sweetener, and black pepper, whisking while heating on medium for about 10 minutes. Remove from heat and serve.

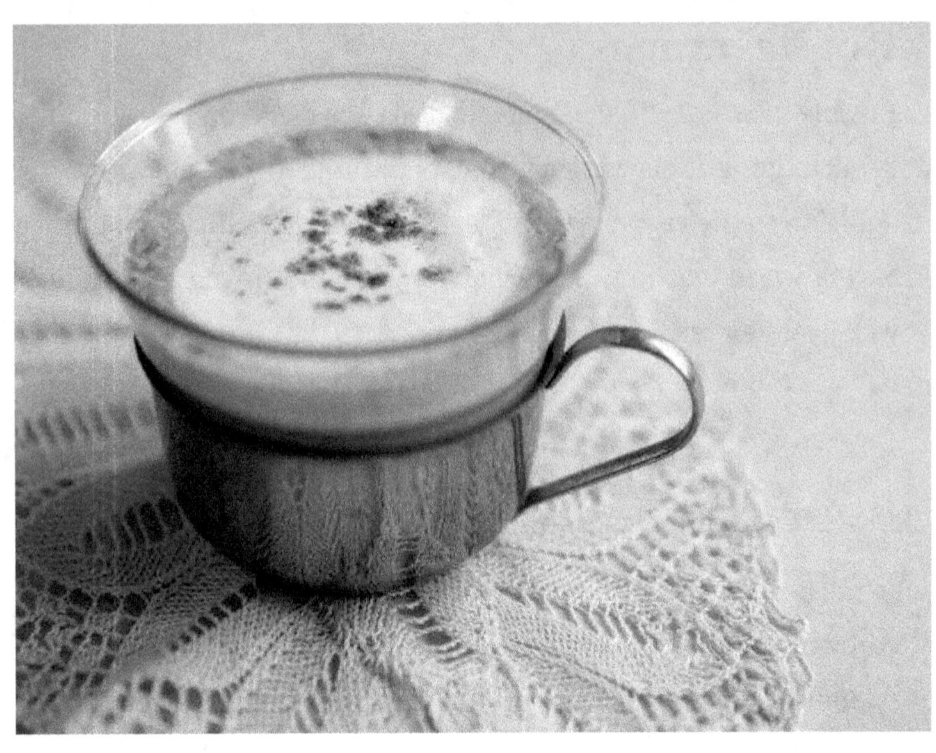

Matcha Milk Tea

Matcha green tea powder has become popular in Asian bakeries as the main ingredient in many pastries, cakes, and puddings. This strain of green tea contains as much, if not more, antioxidants than many fruits and vegetables. Matcha powder is often found in specialty stores and becoming more common in supermarkets with a wide selection of international products and foods.

- 2 cups of almond or coconut milk
- 2 teaspoons of maple syrup or low carb sweetener
- 2 tablespoons matcha green tea powder

Heat the two cups of almond or coconut milk in a saucepan while stirring in the matcha powder and sweetener. Whisk while bringing the milk close to a boil, without boiling the milk, then remove and cool slightly before pouring into a mug to serve.

Mocha Almond Milk

Warm almond milk is whisked with the flavors of freshly ground coffee and cocoa powder. All the ingredients are combined in a small saucepan.

- 1 tablespoon of finely ground coffee beans
- 2 tablespoons of cocoa powder
- 2 cups of coconut or almond milk
- 1 teaspoon of vanilla or almond extract
- 2 teaspoons of maple syrup or low carb sweetener

In a small saucepan, heat the milk and whisk in the coffee grinds and cocoa powder. Stir vigorously with a whisk, then add in the vanilla or almond extract, and sweetener. Serve warm and top with a light dusting of cocoa powder. For a stronger chocolate flavor, melt ½ cup of dark baker's chocolate in the milk instead of cocoa powder. Cinnamon is another great topping to add when serving this drink.

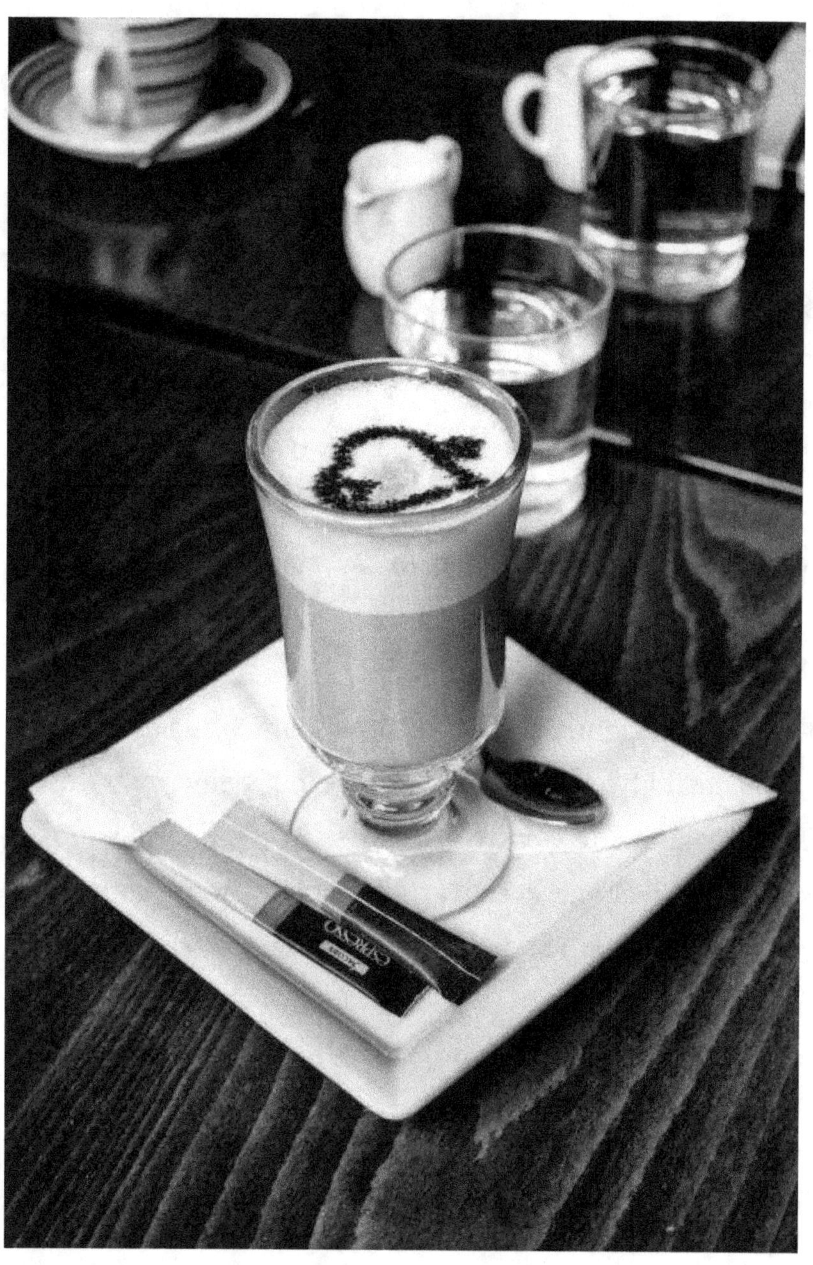

Masala Chai Milk Tea

Masala chai is a fragrant and spicy tea that can be found in some tea shops as a loose-leaf, or in some grocery or natural food stores in tea bags. Either option can be used for the preparation of this drink.

- ½ cup of loose-leaf masala chai (or two tea bags of chai)
- 2 cups of coconut or almond milk
- 2 teaspoons of maple syrup or raw sugar
- 1 teaspoon of vanilla extract (optional)

Heat the milk and gently stir in the loose-leaf masala chai tea. If not available, add two tea bags and drape the strings over the side of the cooking pot. Gently stir in the sweetener and almond extract. Reduce heat and keep warm for at least 10 minutes before serving. This will allow the masala chai to steep longer and strengthen the flavor.

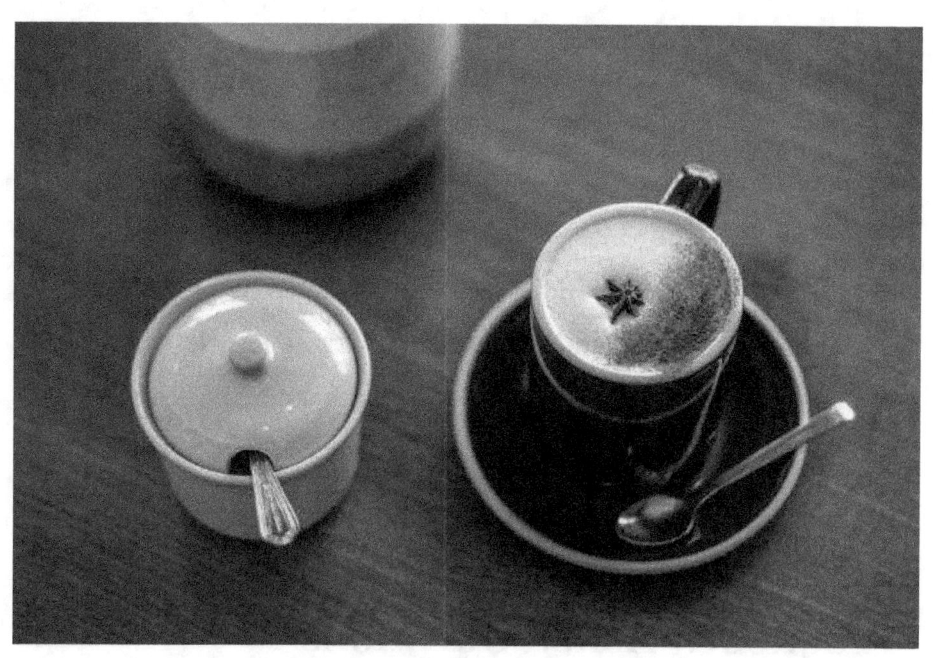

Chapter 9: Conclusion

Adapting to a plant-based diet takes practice and patience, though in time you'll benefit from the changes to your food choices and notice the effects better eating has, including weight loss, prevention, and treatment of chronic conditions and diseases, while maintaining a healthy diet and lifestyle.

Frequently Asked Questions

Do you have any questions or lingering thoughts on the plant-based diet and how to make it work best for you? If you're new to starting your journey on a vegan diet, there may be a lot of questions as you begin trying new foods and combinations of flavors. Some foods, like tofu, may take a while to get used to if you're not accustomed to the texture and how this superfood absorbs many flavors. Cooking with miso and trying new fruits and vegetables may also seem ...

Question: How Long Will It Take to Get Used to Eating Only Vegan or Plant-Based Foods? Should I Make the Switch All at Once or in Stages?

Answer: It takes a month or two to get used to a vegan diet, at least on average, though this varies considerably based on each individual case. If you generally eat a lot of vegetables and plant-based foods already, with little dairy or meat, the transition to plant-based eating won't feel extreme. For heavy meat-eaters, there is a bit more of a "shock", and for this reason, it's best to make changes gradually, by reducing meat and dairy portions while increasing the addition and portions of more fruits, vegetables, nuts, and seeds. Some people are hesitant to try certain foods, like tofu or a new vegetable or fruit, for example, it's best to experience a meal prepared in a restaurant with this item included, to gain a more positive idea about its taste and usefulness. Fortunately, there are a growing number of restaurants that serve only vegan or plant-based foods, while many mainstream eateries offer many vegan dishes and alternatives to meat and dairy options. The more adventurous you become with trying new foods, the more you'll learn to enjoy plant-based eating, and while you may not like everything you try, there will be some new foods worth adding to your weekly shopping list.

Question: Is There a Risk of Eating Too Many Nuts or Seeds?

Answer: Unless you have an allergy or food sensitivity, there is generally no risk involved with enjoying lots of nuts and seeds, and chances are, you'll only eat a few at a time, as they satisfy an appetite relatively well. If you are concerned about food sensitivity, it's best to check with a doctor or medical professional for allergy tests to confirm. If there is an allergy to certain types of nuts, you may still have the option of enjoying a wide range of seeds (pumpkin, squash, sunflower, sesame seeds, etc.). There are some products on the market that aim to provide peanut-free or nut-free options, though it's best to check if there are ingredients to avoid, such as dairy, high levels of sodium and/or sugar and artificial flavors.

Question: If I Only Choose One or Two Fruits Each Week as Part of My Grocery List, Which Fruit Options Are the Best in Terms of Nutrients That I Should Consider?

Answer: All fruit is beneficial, and any variety can be chosen as part of your regular shopping trip. It also depends on the types of nutrients you wish to increase in your diet, and which deficiencies you aim to avoid. For example, bananas are an excellent source of potassium, which is great for reducing water retention. If you want to increase the antioxidant amount in your diet, consider strawberries, cherries, blueberries, raspberries, blackberries, and currants. Apples and citrus fruits are excellent sources of vitamin C. All fruits, in general, are great for providing a high dose of fiber that is beneficial for everyone.

Question: Is There a Vegan Substitute for Every Meat and Dairy Food Item?

Answer: Currently, there appears to be a non-animal product version for everything, though some brands or options may be preferred over others. If you're new to the world of dairy and meat-alterative products, this will take time to learn the different options and determine which are the best for you. For example, some products may contain additives, while others are more natural with fewer preservatives. Some brands of tofu are better than others. Read labels, ingredients, and reviews on products to get a better idea of what's available.

Question: Is It More Expensive to Eat a Plant-Based Diet, Especially If You Choose the Best Quality Foods, Such as Organic and Local?

Answer: Sometimes, certain foods and products will cost more for better quality. This is basically the same principle for all diets, with or without meat and dairy. If budgeting is a concern, consider buying as many foods fresh or frozen (without additives) as possible, and avoid specialty or artisan versions of different foods, as they tend to be pricier and don't enhance your diet any further. Sticking with a basic assortment of foods is the best way to ensure that you'll have all the nutrients you need for a healthy diet, without breaking your budget or buying unnecessary items.

Questions: Do I Need to Take Supplements on a Vegan Diet?

Answer: Some people require supplements if they cannot eat certain foods, and must increase the number of nutrients they have in their diet, to avoid deficiencies. This would apply to anyone who cannot eat nuts or soy products, due to allergies, or must avoid certain fruits and vegetables for the same reason. If omitting certain foods means lacking in a nutrient, it may be found in other sources of protein or fiber, for example, such as chia seeds, though a supplement is a way to guarantee no deficiencies will occur as a result.